T0317055

Thieme

To Paul Hammer, my beloved son

The Patient—Practitioner Relationship in Acupuncture

Leon I. Hammer, MD
Chairman of the Governing Board
Dragon Rises College of Oriental Medicine
Gainesville, Florida
USA

Thieme
Stuttgart · New York

Library of Congress Cataloging-in-Publication Data is available from the publisher.

Artist: Jaqueline Bühler, Basel, Switzerland.
Jacq.buehler@vtxnet.ch
Cover: "Von einem zum andern"
(From one to the other)
p. 5: "Die Unzertrennlichen" (Inseparable)
p. 83: "Harmonisches Paar"
(Harmonious couple)

© 2009 Georg Thieme Verlag,
Rüdigerstrasse 14, 70469 Stuttgart,
Germany
http://www.thieme.de

Thieme New York, 333 Seventh Avenue,
New York, NY 10 001, USA
http://www.thieme.com

Cover design: Thieme Publishing Group
Typesetting by Ziegler + Müller,
text form files, Kirchentellinsfurt, Germany
Printed in Germany by Offizin Andersen
Nexö Leipzig GmbH, Zwenkau

ISBN 978-3-13-148841-1   1 2 3 4 5 6

Important note: Medicine is an ever-changing science undergoing continual development. Research and clinical experience are continually expanding our knowledge, in particular our knowledge of proper treatment and drug therapy. Insofar as this book mentions any dosage or application, readers may rest assured that the authors, editors, and publishers have made every effort to ensure that such references are in accordance with **the state of knowledge at the time of production of the book.**

Nevertheless, this does not involve, imply, or express any guarantee or responsibility on the part of the publishers in respect to any dosage instructions and forms of applications stated in the book. **Every user is requested to examine carefully** the manufacturers' leaflets accompanying each drug and to check, if necessary in consultation with a physician or specialist, whether the dosage schedules mentioned therein or the contraindications stated by the manufacturers differ from the statements made in the present book. Such examination is particularly important with drugs that are either rarely used or have been newly released on the market. Every dosage schedule or every form of application used is entirely at the user's own risk and responsibility. The authors and publishers request every user to report to the publishers any discrepancies or inaccuracies noticed. If errors in this work are found after publication, errata will be posted at www.thieme.com on the product description page.

Foreword

The sage healers of ancient times were able to heal the heart of humanity, and thus prevent disease from arising. Today's doctors only know how to treat disease when it has already manifested in physical form, and don't know anymore how to work with the heart. This situation can be compared to the process of pruning tree branches while neglecting the tap root, or to working downstream without awareness of the properties of the wellspring. Is this not an ignorant way to go about the business of medicine? If you wish to bring about real healing, you must first and foremost treat a person's heart. You must bring the heart on the right path, so that it can be filled and sustained by a universal sense of truth. You must get it to a place where it can safely abandon all doubting and worrying and obsessing in senselessly looping patterns, where it can let go of any anxiety provoking imbalances, and where it is willing to surrender all "me, me, me" and all "this is his/her fault!" Try and awaken the heart to acknowledge and regret all the wrong that one has done, to lay down all selfish attachments, and to trans-form one's small and self-centered world for the glorious universe wherein we are all one, and wherein there is nothing to do but praise its existence. This is the master method of the enlightened physician—healing through the heart. Or, in different words from the ancient record: the enlightened doctor intervenes before physical disease manifests, while the average physician springs into action only after disease has become apparent. To treat before this stage, this is the terrain of healing the core—the heart; to treat afterwards, this is the realm of dietary therapy, herbal therapy, acupuncture, and moxibustion. Although there are these two types of therapeutic paths, there is really only one core law of healing: All dis-ease comes from the heart.

Thus the 16th century Korean master physician Hur Jun synthesizes a lifetime of clinical insight on the importance of treating the heart in *Dongyi baojian*

(Precious Reflections by an Eastern Physician). I can think of no better quotation to introduce this modest yet vitally essential volume by Leon Hammer.

Today as during the time of Hur Jun, the profession of Chinese medicine has become a technique-oriented métier. Dr. Hammer's book on the client–practitioner relationship in acupuncture, therefore, may strike us as the personal musings of an accomplished psychiatrist turned Chinese medicine practitioner that are not directly related to the mainstream of our field. Nothing could be further from the truth. As with his classic publications on Chinese medicine psychology and pulse diagnosis, *The Patient–Practitioner Relationship in Acupuncture* is the work of a seasoned clinician who transmits with great urgency and trademark humility the virtues, skills and attitudes that are indispensable for any genuine engagement with the timeless art of Chinese medicine.

While Dr. Hammer has repeatedly demonstrated his generosity to younger generations of Chinese medicine practitioners by relating his clinical knowledge and experience in prolific detail, this volume exhibits more of a *zen*-like quality. The reader finds a booklet by a wise and compassionate physician who describes with great clarity and simplicity the essentials of his craft, in this case the sacred space of the client–practitioner interaction. Wu Tang, the 18th century compiler of Fever School therapeutics, once wrote of this essence in the preface of his landmark *Wenbing tiaobian* (Systematic Differentiation of Warm Diseases): "Medicine is the way of compassion–led by wisdom and humility, assisted by courage, and completed by compassion." By transmitting and palpably modeling to us the unassuming quality of a traditional Chinese medicine saint, Leon Hammer reminds all of us of the deep commitment that brought us to this profession in the first place—the desire to care for others, in the most whole and complete way possible. For me, this book represents an authentic echo of Sun Simiao's 7th century description of the great physician (*Dayi jingcheng*):

The great physician serves to live in harmony with nature, and teaches his patients to do the same. He will stay calm and completely committed when treating disease. He will not give way to personal wishes and desires, but above all else hold and nurture a deep feeling of compassion. He will be devoted to the task of saving the sacred spark of life in every creature that still carries it. He will strive to maintain a clear mind and be willing to hold himself to the highest standards. He will consider it to be his sacred mandate to diagnose sufferings and treat disease. He will not be boastful about his skills and not driven by the greed for material things. Above all, he will keep an open heart. As he moves on the right path, he will receive great happiness as a reward without asking for anything in return.

Heiner Fruehauf, PhD
Founding Professor
School of Classical Chinese Medicine
National College of Natural Medicine
Portland, Oregon

Preface

This book for acupuncturists on the therapeutic relationship is not focused on pathology; only on the issues we encounter with other human beings, none of whom is without some part of themselves that is a problem to them as well as to others.

Acupuncturists may question the need to read a work on the therapeutic relationship. After all, by law they are only required to make a Chinese Medicine diagnosis, prescribe herbs, and place the needles in appropriate acupuncture points. This is their legal "scope of practice." The "Traditional" Chinese Medicine model arising from mainland China discourages encountering people on any platform other than one that involves inserting needles, dispensing herbs, and allied techniques such as massage, exercise, and nutrition. Emotional issues, with rare exceptions, are referred out.

However, acupuncturists work with people, not charts or manikins. And people who work with "energy" have a special obligation to consider all of the implications that enter into the transfers of energy between the specific role of the therapist and the role of the patient.

While the implementation of some of the principles in this book may require at times a referral to a more professionally trained psychologist, the principles themselves are necessary ingredients in the successful encounter between any two human beings. This is especially true if one is "helping" and the other is being "helped." My goal is not to teach psychotherapy, but to enhance the practitioner's propensity and innate talent to heal.

When practitioners make any form of contact with someone seeking help, they have entered into a therapeutic relationship that inevitably involves all of the contents of this book. Those who think otherwise do so at their own risk, and do so even more at the patient's risk. There is no escape from this reality in the successful practice of this profession.

Leon I. Hammer, MD

Acknowledgments

With regard to the subject of this book I am especially grateful to Augusta Schlesinger, PhD, a courageous 76-year-old woman who made a remarkable metamorphosis from retired housewife to become the founder of the Bureau of Child Guidance in the New York City school system and courts. She was my first therapist from 1946 until her death in 1951. She is the model for the content of this book.

I also owe a deep debt of gratitude to the William A. White Institute of Psychiatry and Psychoanalysis in New York, where I received my psychoanalytic training, and to my teachers Clara Thompson, MD, Gerard Chernowski, MD, Eric Fromm, PhD, Ernst Schactel, PhD, Harry Bone, PhD, Harry Stack Sullivan, MD, Florence Powdermaker, MD, Asya Kadis, PhD, Anina Brandt, PhD, Ana Gourevitch, PhD, and Ralph Crowley, MD.

I am also indebted to Alexander Lowen, MD, John Pierakos, MD (bioenergetics), and to Fritz Perls, MD (gestalt therapy), all of whom I studied with in my post-psychoanalytic training.

For the present I am grateful to Pamela Smith, AP, and Hamilton Rott, AP, who made helpful suggestions; to Candice Nelms who wrote an introductory sheet for the publisher; and to all those who over the years challenged me to answer their questions.

I also wish to acknowledge Jaqueline Buehler, a Swiss artist, for her generosity in contributing her marvelous sculptures for the cover and the section openers of this little book.

I am grateful to Thieme for accepting this book for publication, and most of all I wish to acknowledge Angelika Findgott's sensitive and intelligent guidance in this project, for which I am endlessly grateful. As my editor she made this process a joy, and her creativity turned a rough manuscript into a highly readable and well-organized book. Thank you.

Table of Contents

Section II—Questions and Answers

Introduction

The following book for acupuncturists on the therapeutic relationship is presented with the intention of avoiding psychological jargon as far as possible. Therefore, words such as transference, counter-transference, and resistance are avoided, and the information is offered in everyday language. I will refer to the acupuncturist-therapist as "therapist" or (Chinese Medicine—CM) "practitioner."

According to the dictionary[1] "therapy" is defined as the "remedial treatment of mental or bodily disorder … designed or serving to bring about rehabilitation or social adjustment." However, therapy also involves a healing interaction with other living beings, for which there are universal precepts for relationships, which are covered in the following chapters.

There is also an inevitable amount of repetition since many subjects such as empathy and intuition overlap. Let us celebrate the lack of rigid organization and the dividend of reiteration as a blessing rather than a curse, since it is with repetition that we learn.

I have organized the book into two sections. The first section covers the basic tenets of a therapeutic relationship independent of context, and is based upon my training and experience as a psychiatrist-psychoanalyst. Having practiced both Chinese Medicine and psychiatry-psychoanalysis, I can categorically assert that the problems encountered in each are essentially the same even if the presentations seem widely different.

The second section of the book applies specifically to issues that confront acupuncturists in particular and is drawn from questions elicited from practitioners and students of acupuncture and from my own experience. In this regard, one necessary stabilizing guide throughout all the emotional maelstroms that an acupuncturist may encounter in the therapeutic relationship is their CM diagnosis and the management intervention. Throughout the often confusing and chaotic presentations that patients may make from appointment to appointment, the one steady and enduring quotient will be the CM formulation, which will include, for example, a diagnosis and plan to address the cause of the chaos that threatens the practitioner's objectivity and the therapy. That operational concept and its application should be the practitioner's central focus while he or she applies all that follows in this book to maintaining a working relationship.

In my work, I have experienced both failures and successes. Looking back, especially on the failures, I can see that I have been blessed with the ability to carry on, for which I take no credit and for which I am eternally grateful. Not all of us are so blessed and it is my good fortune to express that gratitude by trying to help others do the same.

General Remarks About the Therapeutic Relationship

The therapeutic relationship has gained recognition as one ineluctable facet of any program attempting to relieve deeply troubled people of their pain and help them to redirect their lives. It is a sympathetic confrontation; a situation in which two human beings work together to remove, for one of them, a critical impasse in their life. Inevitably, both participants are the beneficiaries of this working relationship.

It is also a means of conserving human life; thus, it follows the humanistic tradition. We offer it in distinct opposition to two other traditional ways of dealing with society's "wounded": to destroy them, or to ignore them. The latter is, perhaps, the more common way, and as brutal as the first, for nothing, not even hate, is so much the antithesis of love as apathy; nothing so disheartening to the struggling individual.

The therapeutic relationship takes an optimistic view of human beings, cherishes their potential and the innate drive to realize themselves at their best. Theology, psychology, and the healing arts all direct human beings to psycho-spiritual growth.

We all begin life with a series of fantasies that we are compelled to test despite the wisdom of those who would gainfully advise us otherwise. The best you the practitioner can do is evoke and listen to these fantasies. Your gentle responses will be ignored at first, but not forgotten. They will not be discarded until they have been tested in the laboratory of life. That is one reason why the therapeutic relationship may be discontinuous as a patient suffers through one delusion after another, seeking help when each experiment fails and he or she is strong enough to try the next. You cannot stop the process; only become a resourceful part of it.

Furthermore, the patient comes with the expectation that you will make it possible for them to continue the lifestyle that has made them ill without paying the consequences. The ability to make a connection between the presenting problem and a lifestyle is within the scope and skill of the practitioner, and the remainder of this book will help you make it possible. You encounter a person at an impasse, in a vicious conceptual cycle that leads nowhere except to pain, and at each stage the problem must be conceptually reframed to break that cycle and move on to a greater truth. This person wishes only to stay "intact" while they maintain life-giving "contact," as will be explained in this book and elsewhere.[2] In the following chapters are guidelines to forming and maintaining the bond necessary to achieve the goal of providing life-giving "contact," while breaking the cycle of pain and moving on to a new fulfilling reality.

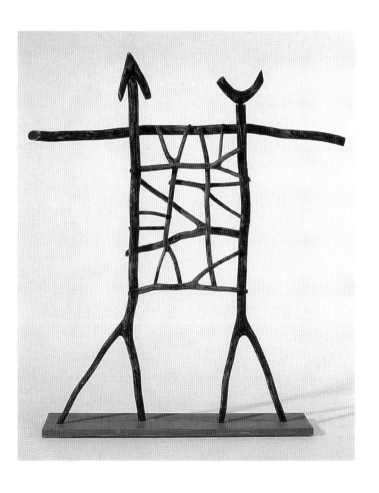

Section I

1   Basic Conditions or Tenets—An Overview

Respect

As we will see below in some detail, respect is the foundation of any successful relationship and foremost in our considerations of a therapeutic relationship. Just as the essence of a therapeutic relationship is contact, so the essence of that contact is the therapist's respect, profound and unequivocal, for the person who depends on them. The mark of a civilized human being, we know, is the respect with which they treat the "weak." This is because respect is the basis of feelings of worth, self-esteem, and trust. A person who is respected comes to respect him- or herself; and when respect for another person is required from them, they begin to know that they have a place in the world, and to see themselves as part of a whole.

Example

A young woman was raised with the notion that she would stay with her parents until death. Not respected as a growing adult, discouraged from normal social relations, not even conscious of her own need to explore and develop socially, she retreated into a grandiose celestial love affair with Christ (a personal affair whose intimate details she was too embarrassed ever to reveal). At 23, she dressed like a dowager. Her parents built an extension to the house for her to live out her life in relative seclusion. She became increasingly depressed and frightened.

Only when she began treatment and saw that the therapist regarded her with respect as an intelligent, capable, and attractive young woman, did she abandon her grandiose phantom love affair and give up her special tie to Jesus. She was also able to give up the intellectual pretensions that were part of her role as her parents' ideal little girl. Once accorded proper respect, freed of her parents' demands, and freed from her compensatory affair with the Lord Jesus, she was able to develop naturally. She abandoned grandiosity, got as job as a waitress, was efficient and charming, and began to lead a life appropriate to her age. She finally left home and associated with people her own age, making a life of her own.

Respect is tested repeatedly, in life and in the therapeutic situation by people who we either do not like or who antagonize us. Some people have a talent for arousing hostility by their words or actions, by their lack of consideration or thoughtlessness. How do we deal with these people? In life we have the option of avoiding these people, and in therapy we have the option of referring them to others when we fail to retain respect, despite all efforts to separate the offensive aspects of their being from those we can gainfully work with.

First, we must admit to ourselves and allow ourselves the full range of our negative reactions, and if necessary we must share them with others—colleagues and supervisors—a subject that we will discuss in more detail later (and always mindful of confidentiality). After venting one's anger to oneself and others we must identify the offending behavior to the "patient" in the context of the positive aspects of his or her being.

Example

A patient repeatedly made inappropriate remarks to teachers, peers, and to his acupuncturist, offending everyone. He seemed to know the exact thing to do or say at the moment when it could do the greatest damage and arouse the greatest response.

This obviously lonely person was able to obtain attention as a child by irritating his parents, who otherwise ignored him. Maintaining "contact" with significant others is a basic requirement for survival when one is most vulnerable. In order to stay "intact," he resorted to a strategy that achieved contact and attention at home, but that did not work outside his family circle.

He criticized my appearance, my surroundings, my work, my voice, and almost every other aspect of my being at one time or another. The closest he came to causing me to terminate the relationship was when he criticized my ethnic background. While agreeing that I could improve in all the directions he attacked, I pointed out that my improvement, except in how I could help him, would be of no benefit for resolving his problems. In addition, he would alienate anyone similarly treated outside of a therapeutic relationship.

His barrage of criticism obscured his positive attributes. He was obviously intelligent and respected, if not liked, for his work as a physicist. His keen observation of all my faults indicated a highly developed awareness, and I wondered if this could be put to good use in the world. He was encouraged to develop an interest in bird-watching, at which he excelled. We very gradually separated the behavior from the intention and concentrated on new strategies to obtain the "contact" without the isolating offensive behavior that elicited a negative response.

In order to undertake this work, respect did not require me to "like" this person. It was necessary for me to identify the positive and to continue to separate it from the destructive in a working relationship he was also engaged in. It was necessary to be more concerned with respect for him than for his respect for me. I would not have accomplished anything for either of us if, like others, I had simply responded with hostility in order to deflect his offensive, often enraging, behavior.

I realize that a practitioner of Chinese Medicine (CM) is not trained to take on the working through of such a project. However, the basic principles must be understood in the context of clinical practice so that it can endure long enough to yield results. Treating the basics of a CM diagnosis will go a long way to facilitating the patient's unraveling of their psychological dilemma if their issues include a "closed heart" or "phlegm misting the orifices" among other things. The needles engender awareness and the breaking of vicious cycles of emotion and energetics.

To continue our discussion of respect, respect also implies **authenticity, objectivity, consistency, commitment**, and **confidentiality**. We shall consider each in turn.

Authenticity

Authentic behavior and communication require directness, honesty, and clarity. If these honest feelings are perceived as critical, we may be afraid that people will identify us as "not so nice" that we may be rejected and/or attacked. Clearly, then, authenticity, directness in human communication, is only possible for people with a "self" that is not dependent upon external approval for its existence.

Directness and Disapproval

We live in a culture that does not allow us to be ourselves. The corporate world we are dominated by admires individuality in the abstract but discourages it in practice. Ours is not the Jeffersonian society of small, independent entrepreneurs and farmers who could afford to be themselves. In today's world, living with disapproval is a much greater challenge than ever before.

We tend, therefore, to avoid directness, because directness often leads to conflict. Today, this is especially apparent in parent–child relations. Parents seem to be afraid of an open confrontation with a child and of living with the child's anger. We seem to be afraid of anger in general, in all of our relationships, as if the expression of anger were dangerous.

Example

The following is an example of indirect communication, in the form of a mixed message. A young man came to the acupuncturist with his mother. She repeatedly urged him to speak up, to say what was on his mind. Yet, whenever he did this, she interrupted to tell him that she knew that this was not what he thought, that she knew what he was thinking better than he did. This mother was frightened by her son's withdrawal, but even more afraid of his criticism. In order to draw him out, she encouraged him to express himself, but he had learned long before that there was no audience for the "real him," so he withdrew.

Authentic behavior here would have been simply for the mother to acknowledge that her son was not free to think for himself, that she could not bear criticism. That kind of honesty prevents confusion and, at its best, is the modus of change and growth in a relationship, as well within.

Fear of Anger

The problem of anger is perhaps more complex. In only one generation we have moved away from open support for brutality to children (in schools and homes). Instead, we have tended to veer in the other direction, and have come to fear and hide our hostility with a veneer of nicety and political correctness that places us out of touch with ourselves. In such a short time, we do not yet trust ourselves to have learned to express hostility without being destructive. Lack of contact with our hostility has made it assume monstrous proportions, as does anything we hide under a rug. It is true of the human mind that whatever escapes our direct scrutiny becomes fantastic. We have only fantasy or reality from which to choose. Of course, when the expression of one feeling—anger in this instance—is avoided, others such as tenderness are also muted; then mutuality and authenticity in relationships are accordingly and commensurately compromised.

The daily work of tempering fantasy with reality is essential labor in the therapist's own development. The arduous task of learning to live with disapproval and retain belief in oneself is also essential to their function. He or she is often the first and only humanely honest person the patient may ever know; the only model of authenticity they will ever encounter. Authenticity most often becomes an issue in the therapeutic relationship situation when the practitioner is required to confront the patient with feelings or opinions that may provoke anger and conflict. How directly the practitioner does this, without attack or derogation, is of critical importance to their developing relations.

Honesty and Manipulation

We can observe manipulative behavior, the antithesis of honesty and authenticity, at all levels of human intercourse. The manipulative person flatters, lures, misrepresents, deceives, bullies, and threatens—all in order to make someone else act in a certain way. The manipulator makes the object of the maneuvers feel used. Children who are treated this way grow to regard themselves as worthwhile only if they are being used, and will come to fear that if they cease to be useful, they will be discarded. Their insecurity will bring with it resentment and a sense of humiliation, both sources of self-hatred. With manipulation, the medium of transaction is never love, respect, or meaningfully worked-through conflict; it is always a kind of bribe, a kind of submission for a price, a buying and selling of people. Manipulation destroys trust; in children it prevents the development of trust.

And the manipulator, too, suffers. It is not only that their behavior expresses a profound insecurity, but also—because they must have what they want at any cost, including the cost of real ties to people—those ties are precisely what their maneuvers cost them. One usually cannot have both: what one wants *and* the love and respect of those who one must use to get it. Usually, one has to make the choice. Often it is love or loyalty that manipulators seek, and that is always what they lose. To be loved, one must give others a free choice.

Authenticity Recapitulated

Again, the practitioner expresses authenticity with alertness to, immediacy of response to, and willingness to face, the patient's negative feelings directly (which may be indirectly expressed in mannerisms, attitudes, behavior, or in an overt counterattack). By "immediacy" I mean eye contact and touch, the most direct and revealing forms of human interaction. Words are necessary but are easily used and perhaps most often used to obfuscate rather than clarify.

It is easy to avoid these confrontations, but to do so renders the practitioner useless. To do so is to repeat the patient's past experience. That is very far from our goal of offering resources for a new experience and a new model of reality.

Objectivity

By this term we mean the ability to understand the other person's behavior; to understand it as it affects them, as distinct from how it affects us; to understand the need to keep these separate. Its antithesis is egocentricity—the tendency to see everything only as it affects us.

Objectivity makes further demands upon us. It requires that we examine our own values, attitudes, and behavior (in the interest of our constant effort to maintain contact, to be a human "tranquilizer"). Objectivity requires that we weigh our position honestly with regard to the patient. How willing are we to let people depend on us? How willing are we to extend ourselves in the face of resistance, of anger, and of contempt? Can we take the initiative, show that we care about relations with someone who may seem to have little to give in return, who may hardly seem to appreciate our efforts?

Can we honestly consider how much we need to win, especially with younger people? Can we recognize our own stereotypes and prejudices? Can we set them aside in order to seek out and expose another person's need and ability to love? Can we accept this love, however tentatively it is offered, in the spirit in which it is offered? Conversely, can we accept rejection, albeit temporary, without ourselves being set back emotionally? Can we let others near us emotionally? Can we be honest with ourselves, and open with others, about our own fears and hang-ups in order that another person may let us into their life and give us their trust? Questions such as these arise endlessly in human relations and cannot all be anticipated in this context. They must be sought out and faced as they arise.

Consistency and Commitment

Closely related concepts, consistency, and commitment are central to our ability and willingness to stay with a patient through difficult periods, to persist rather than give up. That we are consistent means that we will be reliable, that we can be counted on, that we are not erratic and not unpredictable. That we are committed means that we regard this work, this developing relationship with the patient, as a trust; that we have made a firm decision to stand by them.

When patients realize that the practitioner regards them as worth the struggle necessary for their healing, and stands by them when their problems are most acute or difficult, the experience will accrue to their own self-worth. It is a fundamental prerequisite to self-esteem to be genuinely esteemed by others for one's real self. People who have never been acknowledged and liked for their real selves never cease, throughout their lives, either to seek approval or to avoid disapproval, or both. True self-esteem arising from the esteem of a significant other early in life, or in the context of a therapeutic relationship, obviates the need later for constant reinforcement from either within or without.

The experience is also a potential learning situation for those patients whose tendency is to flee from difficulties. From the steady, consistent commitment and support of the therapist, patients will learn by repeated example to break the old pattern. They will slowly discover that consistently standing their ground in the face of trouble is a viable alternative to running away.

Example

A patient was labeled as crazy by her family and threatened with commitment to a hospital whenever she took a step they found objectionable. Originally an orphan, she felt alone in the world and was uncertain whether she was sane or mad, competent or incompetent. She also now felt acutely the real threat of losing her children and her freedom. A crisis arose when she attempted to take an independent attitude. In the face of her family's efforts to intimidate her and to break her spirit, the therapist gave his consistent support and sustenance. The experience of his commitment to stand fast for her, rather than collapsing before the seemingly inexorably dominating family, became the basis for her to withstand further pressure from her family.

This patient came to know herself as a person of substance as she experienced her own power within a family whose domination collapsed when it was challenged, as happens with most bullies. For her, it has led to more equal relationships with other people.

Confidentiality

As a matter of respect, this term speaks for itself. Our obligation is to maintain confidentiality, except for matters of life and death (suicide, or possibly homicide, for example, which might be prevented by intervention). These are issues that touch personal values, and we respond to them accordingly. I explain to patients that I must share such information with other appropriate people, because matters of life and death are too great a responsibility to handle alone.

Perhaps keeping confidence goes against the grain; we are all naturally gregarious and need to share social knowledge, need to talk about people, though we generally derogate that need by calling our talk gossip. When, for the sake of another person, we forego the pleasure, and the relief from tension, that comes from telling secrets, we are in effect giving that person to understand that he or she is special to us. When we give another person's needs precedence over our own, we act in love. This is, ultimately, a profound source of self-esteem for both partners.

Boundaries

Both the subjects of confidentiality and commitment are also involved in a discussion of boundaries. Confidentiality is an obvious boundary. Equally obvious is the extent of our commitment to the life of the patient and of others. As part of our contract (to be discussed in Chapter 4), we inform the patient of the circumstances when we break that confidentiality: matters of life and death, suicide, and homicide.

Beyond those obvious boundary issues is the degree to which the practitioner and the patient are involved in each other's personal lives. Generally agreed is that sexual relationships are completely taboo.

The issue of socializing is where the boundary lines are less clear and are evaluated in terms of the ability of the therapist to maintain objectivity in social situations. Examples include being invited for dinner, to a party, to a movie, or to the theater. The first rule is to engage the patient socially only in a group situation. A young insecure patient, moving to an apartment for the first time, had a house warming to which the acupuncturist was invited. It was not necessary for the acupuncturist to accept this invitation for the work to continue. However, an acceptance was a sign of recognition of the importance of the move and the event to the patient, and of the "heart" aspect of the acupuncturist's involvement.

Readiness for Change

We must distinguish *our* emotional readiness for change from the *patient's*. We cannot expect people to change overnight to act according to what we think is in their best interests if they are not equipped to act.

Above I gave an example under the discussion of "Consistency and Commitment" of a woman who was indoctrinated by her family into believing herself inferior and dependent on them in a way that interfered with her ability to "become" herself. In this example she was encouraged to act only when she was ready.

I was privy to the exigencies of the early years of women's liberation when many formerly dependent middle-aged women with no training in life left their husbands and then foundered. It appears that they often developed deep depression and even life-threatening diseases such as cancer in greater numbers than their peers. They were encouraged to change their lives by activists when they were not ready to do what otherwise might have been for the best.

I cannot attest to the truth of the following but only report what I was told. An acquaintance of mine was a leading member of the feminist movement during the 1970s and early 1980s. We frequently met socially and at least on one occasion professionally. She once told me that she regretted beginning the woman's liberation movement in the way she did, because middle-aged women who had left their husbands were flocking to her with serious mental, emotional, and physical illnesses, including, all too frequently, cancer. In response she felt obligated to set up and support a safe transition house for such women in a nearby town where she provided assistance, both emotionally and medically as well as financially.

In no way is this a criticism of the woman's liberation movement (which I support), just that transitions must be carefully monitored in order to avoid negative consequences. I introduce herbs (and medications) gradually to tolerance levels, and reduce them even more slowly to avoid a shock to the system and a rebound effect.

Expectations

We cannot expect the patient to relate to us without the mental and emotional baggage they carry. People in the healing professions often express dismay that their patients create difficulties for them from the very beginning of their contact. How can a person in distress due to their maladaptive patterns automatically suspend these patterns in the presence of the person they expect assistance from? If we force them to pretend to be otherwise as a condition of our contract with them, what is the purpose of coming to see us and what are we working with? My practice of both psychiatry and acupuncture was built on the referrals from other practitioners who did not wish to deal with "difficult" patients. *All* human beings are difficult.

Generally, the patient's problems reflect mistrust of themselves and others. It is a mistrust often rooted in past experience, experience where being cared for also meant being controlled. It is natural to resent it, even when the need for control from the outside is great, for it violates an individual's need to be his or her own boss. So the patient is caught on the horns of a dilemma: they need our care, but they fear our power over them if they give in to that need. To put it another way: needing contact with us to survive, they simultaneously experience it as a threat to the individuality they naturally cherish.

We must respect this dilemma, and our respect will be another new and helpful experience for the patient. In order that they may choose to make the life-saving contact, we, too, must cherish their individuality, even as we help them to face the shortcomings that have made them so vulnerable.

Values

We come now to the final issue in this discussion of tenets and conditions: the issue of values, of ethical and moral standards and beliefs. The two people in the therapeutic relationship (and in many other situations) are bound to find that their values differ.

Of first importance here is that the therapist must be clear about his or her own values, confusion, uncertainties, and conflicts. What matters here is not that differences exist, nor even what those specific differences are, but that the process of communication goes on, that two people whose values may differ considerably engage in common work in an atmosphere of mutual respect. That respect must come first from the therapist even in the face of disrespect, which while identified as such, is responded to within the context of the patient's limited and often maladaptive methods of making contact.

Judgment of Good and Bad

When we think about values, it is inevitable that we employ terms such as negative and positive, bad and good—terms that imply judgment. They are useful terms, though they are not helpful if used as stigmas or mere labels. For every human situation has positive and negative elements, good and bad aspects. In the therapeutic relationship, we are obliged to separate carefully and clearly identify the positive and negative elements of any particular situation. Our doing so will enable the patient to shift their own identification from the negative, which has been in the foreground of their awareness, to the positive, for which they have been slow to give themselves credit.

Example

A mother constantly worried about her child's health, and hated herself for it, thinking her worry a sign of her inadequacy as a mother (just as her estranged husband thought it a reflection of her general inadequacy). The therapeutic relationship work enabled her to distinguish her healthy, positive concern for her child (the kind that all children need to feel) from those concerns that were unrealistic and exaggerated. Once she distinguished the positive nurturing instinct from the worries stemming from lack of confidence (that she was weak, that she was not sufficiently resilient, that anyone under her direct care must suffer from her deficiencies), those negative issues became available for resolution. Thus, she could draw strength from the positive to face the negative.

In fact, I found as a child psychiatrist, that more often than not, the child who was "overprotected" was known instinctively by the mother to have some significant defect and needed the extra protection. The relief experienced by these vilified mothers when someone recognized their concern as appropriate, changed them and the entire family dynamics. We must always look for the good in what at first seems like all bad.

Guilt and Evil

A discussion of values, of positive and negative aspects of behavior or personality, brings us to guilt, to what people perceive as the "evil" within. We have already said that the negative attributes in people arise originally as a positive, though perhaps misplaced, attempt to make some unbearable life situation more bearable.

"Evil" is originally a miscalculation, not malice aforethought. Maladaptations develop a life of their own if they become the major modus of self-identity. At this stage of the progression, people may be "evil" and experience it as their strength, their power, and their pleasure, while those adversely affected would call it "bad."

If we wish to help someone identify and transform the "evil" in them, we can do so only by first helping them see that this "evil" actually interferes with the deepest satisfactions they seek in life. It will not help if they see merely that this "evil" interferes with anyone else's satisfaction, except that this might ultimately reduce their own. To blame him or her, however, may evoke only guilt. This leads to resentment and a still greater resistance to understanding, because resentment is a negative feeling, which by itself deepens the sense of "evil." Approaching the "evil" in a person as a deterrent to his or her own life, however, leads to insight and, in time, provides motivation for change.

The skill in the therapeutic relationship lies in helping patients discover what they really want, and in helping them see how they keep themselves from getting it.

2 Conditions for Healing, Growth, and Change

Confronting the Best and the Worst

People can grow and change when they face the best and the worst in themselves, with the help of another person. Courage is the currency of this engagement and the example is set by the therapist. This "worst" is a set of early life adaptations that later in life prove to be maladaptive. However, even in the context of the "worst" one can search for and differentiate the "best." The quest for survival is the goal of all behavior, however counterproductive. It evokes talents that, if delineated from the failure, can be the basis of a productive life.

Confronting the Irrational

Without the commitment I referred to in Chapter 1, it is impossible to realize a critical therapeutic principle—that of helping people to become aware of the irrational in themselves. For it is the irrational in people, when it is hidden or expressed only indirectly, that causes problems. The practitioner's job is to bring it out, to uncover what patients fear is crazy inside them, and to release them from this fear; release them so that they may live freely.

Confronting Psychic Pain: Negative and Positive

My value system holds that, in one way or another, we must face pain and experience it as a condition of growth. Indeed, facing one's unhappiness with an involved, attentive other person can itself be a positive new experience. It is also useful to explore the positive aspects of that pain and how through our adaptations pain has stimulated and shaped the strongest aspects of our personality.

This is in sharp contrast to the belief system in our time that holds and encourages the position that it is "cool" to avoid pain. The drug culture began in the post-World War II period with legal tranquilizers encouraged by physicians and drug companies, spreading naturally to the young in the 1960s, who found illegal drugs more effective and appealing than their parents' methods of escape.

These value models must be clearly delineated as different life perspectives and examined in terms of their ramifications as lifestyles, not as good or bad.

Taking a Risk

One of the conditions for healing in a therapeutic relationship is the ability of the practitioner to take a risk. It may be necessary at various times to risk the patient's anger, to risk being wrong, to risk our pride.

For example, frequently in their work, practitioners are faced with the patient's silence. They are obliged to interpret this silence and respond to it—and to take the chance that their interpretation may be wrong, for silence may express many attitudes. It may be that the patient is one of those people for whom speech, or even eye contact, is very difficult. He or she offers no clues, and what he or she intends will depend on the total situation. It may simply be that being quiet and passive in another person's presence, who respects and returns this silence, is for the patient a kind of healing. Or, it may be that the patient's silence is a signal to the practitioner to initiate contact.

A third possibility is that it may be an angry silence that will freeze into obstinate resistance if the practitioner does not challenge it.

In any case, the practitioner uses intuition to interpret and respond. Whether or not to allow the silence to go on and take the risk of not being "helpful," whether or not to take a step toward the patient and risk a rebuff, the practitioner must be willing to accept the risk. He or she must be willing to make a mistake for the sake of the patient, and be willing to adjust his or her behavior accordingly, even to sit in silence for periods of time.

Indeed, the practitioner offers a model of courage to the patient, an act of caring, and a demonstration that one can make mistakes without loss of equilibrium or self-respect. It may be that the demonstration will require a specific admission of error, and even require withstanding the patient's direct attack or indirect attempt to use the occasion to manipulate the practitioner through guilt. That is not important; the practitioner can demonstrate that a person's value and self-respect are not diminished by making errors, and a mistake does not call for derogation or diminished dignity.

With regard to the issue of guilt, one of the most common and virulent forms of manipulation is the claim we make on other people's freedom when they have wronged us in some fashion. If we cannot get what we want from them directly, we use guilt to make them feel they owe us something. Parents do this to control children, and children to control parents; husbands and wives do the same. The patient has, most likely, experienced this form of relating and manipulation through guilt. It is an opportunity to exercise power that the powerless are not easily able to forego.

The practitioner's mistake is an opportunity for manipulation by the patient through guilt. It is very important, therefore, that the practitioner be firm in resisting this maneuver, admit the error, but deny anyone's temptation to abuse him or her because of it. All we owe is an apology, not our integrity. This is extremely important for patients, who will learn, albeit the hard way, to be liberated from their own shackles of guilt and will be freer to live and make mistakes without fear.

Action and Tough Love

Another kind of risk involves action that in one's opinion is in the best interest of the patient and possibly others, but that might evoke severe displeasure in the patient or family.

Example

I am thinking of a young woman I saw in the 1950s whose father was the head of a psychiatric hospital. She was raised in the context of a traditional authoritarian family. She rebelled and tried every aspect of life that was counter to those strict values. Since she was unfamiliar with the world, this rebellion led her to numerous disasters from which she was constantly rescued by her father, who felt his high professional position would be threatened should her troubles become public knowledge. That led to her referral to me.

She made many suicidal gestures that left all concerned in a constant state of dread; her father handled these without her having to take any legal or other consequences. There was always the question about how seriously mentally ill she was, but her father never really wanted to know by hospitalizing her. One weekend night she announced to me by phone that she had taken an overdose. Since there was no 911, I went to her five-floor walk-up, picked up her limp body, carried her down to my car and proceeded to the Bellevue Emergency where she was revived and then hospitalized by me in the psychiatric hospital for a minimum of three weeks, and in that period it was unknown to both of us if this was where she truly belonged. Bellevue hospital, incidentally, was the inspiration for the book and movie called *The Snake Pit*, 1948, starring Olivia de Havilland, who too found herself in an insane asylum. Within days, when the young woman became aware that this would be her fate if she was as insane as she behaved, there was an amazing transformation into sanity that never swerved during the next 20 years that we were in touch. She subsequently moved to Alaska and began a new and productive life.

There are emergencies in which the person is not able to make a choice. When such a choice is necessary for survival, we make it for them in order to preserve life. Likewise, we offer our opinion and state our views about problems and solutions. We do it when it is truly needed. We do it if the person cannot truly do it for him- or herself. We are never entirely certain. We may have to take risks and make mistakes and correct them. At a later time, we must clarify our reasons for taking the choice out of the patient's hands, for taking the initiative, and offer the opportunity to change the survival pattern by an alternative of his or her choice.

For the CM practitioner, these acts of "tough love" that elicit the patient's ire are uncommon. They occur in the context of threatened homicide or suicide, where for the protection of the patient and others the information must be shared, as agreed in the initial contract, and when action may be taken against the patient's will. Here, firmness in the face of the patient's displeasure, as in the example above, is necessary.

Revision of Early Trauma through Positive New Experience

The Conditions

One of the conditions of human growth is having a positive new experience with people dedicated to this purpose. This applies particularly to those aspects of life either neglected or repressed in the past, or shaped by hurtful experience. With this new experience a different self is revealed to the patient from the one they thought themself to be, which was often the one they needed to be to survive, or the one other people needed them to be. The therapeutic relationship must identify the old experience, avoid repeating it, illuminate it, and when the opportunity is present, provide a new experience.

Example

One example is a 50-year-old woman who complained that she felt alive only when she was on stage but was fearful of pursuing the development and professional expression of her specific talent. Instead she escaped into the dominant folds of her husband's strong likes and dislikes, craved food, was endlessly angry, foreswore sex, and felt totally useless. Her ploy, performed partially tongue-in-cheek, was to bring the practitioner "material" (insights, dreams, recollections, problems) and drop it onto his psychological workbench to shape and develop as if she were bringing her shoes to the shoemaker. Inquiry revealed that she had been passively obedient to an ambitious mother, a perfectionist father, and now to a forceful, aggressive husband. Her sense of security depended on a curious dichotomy. In order to be acceptable, she had to be all at once a perfect success, which required enormous drive and self-direction, and an obsequious puppet, which required total passivity. Since outward aggressiveness was an unspoken sin in her family, she chose unconsciously to be the puppet and explode inwardly. This was her maladaptation.

No help would be possible if she had the same experience in the therapeutic relationship situation. I could not allow her to set me up as the authority and herself as the helpless recipient of the products of my "great gifts." She had to work, to explore, to have opinions, to lead the way, to be an authority, and share the responsibility. This was not easy; the maladaptation was corrected only through the necessary new experience of my confidence in her competence to contribute to her own development and my approval of her aggressiveness in her own cause, even with me.

It is a general principle that untoward destructive experience cannot be eradicated but it can be diluted by positive experiences that we encounter from childhood throughout our life from our extended family, from friends, teachers, religious leaders, and in one case, from a sergeant and captain in the army collaborating with me to help a suicidal recruit. I have excerpted the following from a letter that my wife and I recently received from a neighbor's daughter to illustrate:

I think of you both almost daily and thank my lucky stars you came into my life. I have said it before but want to say it again that your influence on me was strong and positive. Thank you (especially to—) for encouraging me to think of myself in ways that were new and different to me, my family, and my peers and thank you to both of you for providing a model of living that was different from every other person I was exposed to as a child.

In the therapeutic relationship as elsewhere, people also need to be known and respected for who they are and not how they can be used. Otherwise, they fail to mature, sometimes lapsing instead into grandiose fantasies that inevitably bring disappointment and unhappiness.

The Results

In the therapeutic relationship situation, all positive experience will foster growth. Negative past experience is impossible to eradicate; however, despite the profound influence of a wounded childhood experience, it can be diluted over time with positive experiences until by proportion it recedes as an influence.

Positive experience will foster growth whether or not it is immediately apparent. We labor in the dark of the immediate and the full consequence of our work is not always obvious. However, if our work is realistic and constructive it will bear fruit and eventually prove worthwhile. And this will be the case even if the therapeutic relationship work is interrupted or prematurely terminated.

The patient, too, may not be able to evaluate the experience until later. They may never, perhaps, be fully aware of its influence. However, even a small, positive interchange with them will enable them to assimilate this encounter, however unconsciously, as a relationship they can return to or upon which they can build new relationships.

3 The Practitioner's Role

Significance

The practitioner is a key figure, the person whose participation enables the patient to see him- or herself and his or her situation in a new and hopefully positive light. This comes about through the process of their close collaboration. What the practitioner does and says makes a difference to the patient. Whatever the contract, for example, "Just treat the pain in my hip," the contact between the practitioner and the patient, the healer and the healed, automatically enters a special realm in which the healer has a special meaning in the life of the person coming for healing. I repeat what I said in the Preface, that people who work with energy have a special obligation to consider all of the implications that enter into the transfers of energy between the specific role of the therapist and the role of the patient.

The fact that the person has come to the practitioner, for whatever reason, is a statement of a desire to "recover." Most people come for relief of pain (physical or mental), for the practitioner to remove symptoms or illnesses that are interfering with their lives without their having to change.

This book is about achieving a relationship in which context a person may feel safe enough to consider and share a pain that is more significant to their complaint than their hip pain. We know that Retained Emotional Pathogens are diverted from vital organs to joints and muscles and are experienced as pain, the relief from which is the original reason for seeking help. It is through this feeling of safety that we help the person to be able to "choose" to deal with the retained emotion.

Recovery from whatever the problem may be, if not spontaneously revealed, is an evolving, subtle, and highly personal process that could involve evocative questions such as "what would your life be without your illness?" and "what would you change about the past and about yourself if you could?"

A Model

Initially, the practitioner's attitudes and demeanor may serve as a model, not for imitation, but by way of example, for we all know that people, especially young people, learn largely by example. How we live our lives with the patient, how we engage with them in this process we call the therapeutic relationship, what "model of reality" we present—these will determine the kind of influence we exert. As we interact and communicate, we offer alternatives (of both attitudes and behavior) to people whose way of life is troubling to them. To the extent that we are emancipated from fanatical and rigid life models, we can offer to others the opportunity to live more freely, not to create robots in our own image, but to open doors to growth and to lend a hand as people pass through them.

In demonstrating the attitudes and behavior of a yet incomplete, imperfect, growing individual willing to take risks for the patient, the practitioner may become a "culture medium" for the patient, creating the conditions that encourage his or her growth, liberated from the fear of failure. The practitioner is a model of the process, not of the end result. He or she is not omniscient, however. Quite the contrary; what the practitioner knows is very limited.

It may be at some point that the practitioner even needs specific help, which they can accept, from their patient. There can be real growth for both of practitioner and patient in such a situation. What comes to mind is the day I began to come down with the flu. A relatively new client with a great deal of talent and very low self-esteem offered a useful remedy, which I accepted as payment for the session. Both of us were helped.

Physician Know Thyself

Because acupuncturists are an essential ingredient of this work, they need to know themselves. They must inquire into their values and how they shift under stress. They need to ask, "Do I respect individual expression more than conformity, rehabilitation more than punishment, the survival of another person more than the enforcement of my own moral standards?"

In asking such questions of themselves, acupuncturists submit to the same process of "self-learning" as the patient; the acupuncturist's investment in self-learning is the critical example he or she sets for those he or she works with. Indeed, the acupuncturist's willingness to be a part of that process together with the patient is essential. It will enable the practitioner to grow as their relationship with the patient grows. And, as they engage in the same process, their mutual effort profiting both of them, the distinction between them will progressively diminish. That is a definition of a good therapeutic relationship.

The processing of information is, of course, highly subjective. The sum total of our life experience is the filter through which all that is received determines our response. That passage may be crystal clear if our life experience has been relatively straightforward. If it has been inauthentic, disrespectful, and uncaring, the passage may be distorted by expectations of the worst. "Good" and "bad" may come our way. Seeing only good is a form of denial. Seeing only bad leads to "shoot first and ask questions afterward."

As a "participant-observer" (Harry Stack Sullivan's term)[1] we are obligated to examine our own filter and to correct, throughout our lives, as many of our distortions as is humanly possible, so that our feeling, thinking, intuition, and empathy will serve as accurate and useful tools for ourselves and our patients.

Winning–Losing: The Power Struggle

It is important that the practitioner does not allow the therapeutic relationship to be a struggle for power. With a patient whose maladaptive patterns of relating are either direct or subtle power struggles, the issue is inevitable.

Power issues involving the ego are inescapable dilemmas for all human beings, except perhaps the saints, and acupuncturists are simply human. Except for a few obvious ones, the forms power issues take are endless and too extensive for discussion in this book.

To whatever extent the practitioner *needs* to succeed, he or she will fail. Here I distinguish between "need" and "want." The patient will sense that "need," and read it as a challenge to engage and defeat, or to escape from. And the engagement can be deceiving until the patient who seems in endless adulation of the practitioner suddenly rejects them. In either case, this becomes a highly destructive struggle that no one can win, perhaps especially destructive to the patient, already unsure of their position in relation to others.

We must enter the relationship without a need to win, even if winning means the success of the therapy. We must be willing to admit our ignorance and our mistake, and we must be willing to concede our vulnerability. For we, too, are human; we, too, have problems and fears. We must not play a game of superiority. We must allow our worth to speak for itself. **In any contest of worth, we will be worthless to our patient. In a demonstration of concern, however, we have an obligation to lead**. We include the patient among our concerns. Our hope is that in time the concern will become mutual, and that eventually the patient will take the initiative in building his or her own relationship with a third person.

However, if you are the sort of person who does "need" to win, if you sincerely feel yourself superior to the patient, if your temptation is to control, dominate, and manipulate others, then, until the problem is reasonably resolved, you should stay out of the therapeutic relationship. And if you are not aware of this about yourself, consistent struggle with or rejection by patients should alert you to considering this as a possible ingredient in your personality.

The Therapeutic Failure and Resolution

An issue related to the need to win is the difficulty of accepting "failure" in the therapeutic relationship situation. At times, it will become obvious that our work is no longer helpful. It is best to face up to that situation, to acknowledge that (for example) the relationship has become stagnant, that it has become destructive (as many dependent relationships do), that it may be temporarily or permanently deadlocked. The best course, then, if no way is found to break the impasse, is separation. Can we accept this without imagining that we have failed? Can we remember, at such times, that the central issue is not our success or failure but the patient's healthy survival? (And it may be that our own survival requires a break; we cannot afford to lose sight of that, either.)

Example

This example illustrates the appropriateness of separation. A patient said that she wanted help, but at every session she complained about coming, suggesting that the practitioner was making her a prisoner. He found it necessary to point out, repeatedly, the discrepancy between her stated wish to work and her negative behavior as soon as work began. On the practitioner's initiative, and in order that he might bring the point home, they parted. Indeed, they parted again and again. The separations recommended by the practitioner enabled her to re-examine her feelings, to perceive them as distortions, and to convince her that she was not, in fact, his prisoner.

In these circumstances, to continue the work without interruption, stalemated as it was, and to avoid the stigma of failure, would have prevented the patient's necessary correction of perception; and it would have created unbearable frustration for the practitioner. Clearly, the needs of both were served by a (temporary) break of contact.

It is appropriate in this situation, as with all problems encountered in practice, to share the problem with an experienced practitioner or with an acupuncturist's training group. In both the practitioner can explore all aspects of the involved issues, including the patient's and their own psychopathology, with its obvious rewards for the practitioner. From the group one is exposed to a broader body of experience and methods of coping with a situation faced universally by the helping professions.

Another course is possible when the practitioner is unable to cope constructively with the therapeutic relationship. He or she can end it by transferring the patient to someone not similarly disturbed by the situation. This kind of flexibility is one of the great potential strengths of the acupuncturists' training group—working together; it makes such transfers possible with minimal damage to the patient.

Example

One member of a group of acupuncturists in a clinic became involved with a family of five, all of whom turned to her for help of one kind or another. Their sheer number and their complex interrelations, jealousies, and competition began to wear her down. She and our group agreed that the assignment had become impossible. We rushed to provide reinforcements since the group was a related entity, familiar with the family's problems and known to the group from the beginning. Some of the family members were transferred to others of our own group of alternative practitioners.

Separation and termination will be discussed in more detail at the end of Chapter 4.

4   Issues Relevant to Any Therapeutic Relationship

The Contract

The person who comes for acupuncture is asking for help, usually with a specific problem. Most often at this juncture in the evolution of acupuncture in the West, it is a physical ailment. However, whether the goal is physical or emotional, in the beginning the acupuncturist should make a spoken contract with the patient, stating specific therapeutic objectives. This contract involves an understanding of time and money considerations involved in reaching that goal.

After that initial contract, the therapeutic relationship can go in one of several directions. In one direction the goal is reached successfully and the contract terminated. The patient may never return. However, even if the result is not perfect, if the respect emphasized over and over in this book is observed by the acupuncturist, the patient will consider returning if a new problem arises. If the acupuncturist's intention is healthy and his or her energies are correctly directed and intersect with the patient's, they will both have gained something ineffable that now bonds them, often unconsciously. This is so even if they never meet again, though sometimes, years later, the acupuncturist will hear from the patient, who has reached a new level of awareness about what has transpired.

The second possibility is that the contracted goal is not reached. The patient is unlikely to consider returning. However, in the context of respect and acceptance, the same appropriate energetic exchange may have been sufficiently beneficial to the patient to set them on a path to healing unknown to both the acupuncturist and patient. In fact, if set off in the right direction, healing goes on beyond the termination of the contract and contact. More rarely, but it has happened, this person will have an epiphany regarding the positive aspects of the experience, and sometimes even communicate that.

The ending of a contract involves all the strong feelings arising from any separation. These are discussed below in general and in particular in the Section II of the book. However, there are two guidelines to follow. The first is to honor the contract and never to lobby the client to extend it unless you both agree that other matters have arisen in the course of your contact to warrant a new contract. This is a fair question to ask as the contract terminates. Second, psycho-spiritual growth should always be an issue that the therapist must always be prepared to introduce into the consciousness of the therapeutic relationship and as part of the contract. If it is not in the practitioner's awareness the opportunity can be lost.

Contact

General

Basic to the therapeutic relationship, as to life, is contact. Contact means communication, touch, touching another. Human beings cannot survive without it. Apart from the uncertain contribution of heredity, human personality is shaped by the nature and by the quality of contact with other people. If the contact is constructive, people are able to cope well with the stresses of life. If it is destructive, people cope poorly or not at all.

How do we define contact in a therapeutic relationship? It means all communication, verbal and non-verbal, that contributes to human growth: the transmission of feeling, sensation, and thought. It is characterized by certain qualities: by sensitive, respectful attention and care. It is characterized also by its form: listening and response. We refer to the qualities of contact as its "how," and to its form as its "what."

We will consider first the "what"—the technical means, the form and craft of the therapeutic relationship. Then we will explore the "how"—the quality of our contact with a patient. Of its two aspects the second, the "how," is primary, but the first, the "what," guides us along ground on which we stand and move as we work. Both can be learned, but the "how" is more subtle.

A cautionary note

As we begin this discussion, let us note that nothing stated here implies that perfection (perfect attitudes, behavior, understanding, or perfect results) is possible. We are talking simply about tendencies, not absolutes.

The Techniques of Contact

Awareness

As practitioners, we learn to develop skills in communication, which we can think of as having three aspects. The first is the reception of the signal, the second the processing of the signal (our interpretation, our comprehension), the third the response to the signal. (Let us keep in mind that we are describing a unitary experience: listening, response, exploration, cooperation, collaboration are one.) Again, there is what we do, and how we do it. Both involve a variety of signals that we give and receive.

Signals may be verbal or non-verbal. The "how" involves non-verbal signals—an empathetic look, a touch, an affectionate gesture—these often mean more to the patient than words, particularly if he or she is a person who distrusts words. The non-verbal signal can represent a giving of oneself in direct and immediate response to the other person's "felt" need.

Total, direct, immediate contact with whatever is in our environment is a gift that few of us are blessed with, and towards which all of us must strive. The talented observers, whose senses and awareness are unfettered by inhibition, or indifference, stand out among us, as do Darwin, Galileo, or Copernicus for example. To be completely in the here and now, with as much of ourselves as possible, is an expression of completeness, satisfaction, and fulfillment. Some of us will be more immediately aware with one or another sensory faculty (in the spectrum that ranges from hearing to intuition). We identify and use the best we have as we live and work. We also simultaneously develop that which lies dormant or undeveloped. Our effort "to be" is the soil in which those who depend on us may also grow. Our purpose, our attitude towards being, and our awareness is the hope on which those in despair may begin to find affirmation of their own being.

I wish to emphasize here that however important our spontaneous aware-ness and intuition (discussed below) of the patient's condition, even enhanced by years of experience, it is not enough on which to base a diagnostic formula-tion and management plan. Working from our instinctive knowledge we are obligated to verify that information with knowledge from other established objective sources in the medicine we practice. I have seen too many instances of practitioners acting only on instinct or studied observation, with tragic out-comes. We must ultimately justify our instinctively driven therapeutic actions firmly on the foundation provided by the proven methodologies of the medi-cine of our choice.

The Different Techniques in Turn

Asking

Asking is one of the four principal methods of knowing in Chinese Medicine (CM). There is a formal aspect to it that is necessary to obtaining the diagnostic data studied and practiced in schools of acupuncture. The patient will provide information within the parameters of what he or she feels comfortable to share with another person. From other diagnostic tools such as the pulse, or from body language, eye contact, voice, and our intuition, we may be aware that our patient is not telling us the entire story. And everyone's life is a story wait-ing and needing to be told.

Here we are concerned with the informal aspect of how we meet that need in a fashion that enhances the therapeutic relationship. Therefore, what we ask for in this context is always considered within the framework of the patient's sensitivities. For example, noticing that something changes in the patient's de-meanor, voice, or color when the subject of children arises, one can approach the subject indirectly by saying: "Wow, you have five children and I am having trouble raising just one," or "You have one child, and one difficult child can feel like 10."

Some people who need to hide their feelings and are threatened by the pos-sibility that others can discern them through ordinary human contact are dis-armed when the observation is made impersonally. For example, if during an interview I say to the patient, "I have the feeling that you are sad" they often respond defensively. However, if I say, "There is a quality on your pulse that indicates that you may be sad," the response in my experience has been a remarkable catharsis. Grown men have broken down and cried in my office.

With some people, the acupuncturist will probably engage their deeper hidden feelings by just "rapping." What is love? What is a friend? What is work, or learning, or one's relation to authority? What is one's place in the world? Who are we, and what about God? We call this rapping, because we alternative practitioners do not have the final answers to these philosophical questions. We can serve as a useful sounding board for others who are looking for thoughtful responsiveness in a permissive, non-dogmatic atmosphere. Often we learn a great deal.

Listening

Content is the most obvious aspect of listening. However, the art of listening involves sensitivity to the relationship between what is being said and how it is being said.

Many years ago, the well-known psychoanalyst, Theodore Reik, wrote a book called *Listening With the Third Ear* in which he delineated those subtle aspects of hearing that he called "listening."[1] What is the purpose of "listening" with the third ear? The object is to reach beyond the obvious to the core, to the nucleus of the person's real self. This is the reality, T.S. Eliot said, that human beings instinctively avoid.

We listen for content: what is the patient talking about—mother, father, girl- or boyfriend, self, work—and we listen to the sound of their voice, for it will convey just as important a message. How do they sound when they talk about their mother, themselves, work? One sound is loud and clear; they have nothing to hide. One sound is high-pitched with fear or quivering with anger and hurt. One sound is too loud; what attitude are they striking? Another sound is too soft, as if to cover up something they do not want to look at. Is the patient's tone of voice consistent with their words, or are they at odds? Can we infer that they are saying one thing and feeling another, something quite antithetical (as will happen if they do not recognize their feelings, or if they fear they will be repellent to the therapist)?

Preoccupation with a particular subject is an important indicator of the central issue that should concern the therapeutic interaction. Drug addicts, for example, inevitably return to this subject as if there is no other subject that matters. On the other hand the key to at least one layer of a person leading to the core can be what is avoided. Frequently, people come and speak for hours about their problems with one parent or person in their life. The sheer repetition of one theme leading nowhere is a signal that this is not the real issue. The drug addict who speaks of nothing else is avoiding the rest of life.

The "five element" school of CM teaches the practitioner to listen for what is usually indirectly expressed in order to identify the phase that is central in the patient's life. Frequently, these signs indicate possible disharmony. In that system, the sound of the voice allows us to identify that phase. The groan is associated with water; the moan with metal; the shout with wood; excessive laughter with fire; and the singsong voice with earth.

Each phase is associated with a different primary issue. For fire we hear or feel that the innermost issue is warmth; for earth it is comfort; for metal it is self-esteem; for water it is reassurance; and for wood it is direction. Though I no longer totally subscribe to the "System of Correspondences," it is instructive as a way of knowing people, their personality, and their problems on all levels of being.

Another system, according to Dr. Shen[2] makes the following normal voice and phase connections, deviations from which indicate disharmony:

Metal	Very strong, loud, and clear, carrying a long distance.
Earth	Stronger than fire, wood, and water with a wide range but less powerful than metal. Many opera singers have this body type and voice.
Fire	High-pitched, loud and sharp.
Wood	Strong though not as strong as metal.
Water	Soft.

"Listening with the third ear" also involves separating the words from the intention or what a person says and what they want. A young woman spoke endlessly about her grief and anger at being left by her husband and yet the thread of her conversation was money and not love.

Feeling

Feeling is another mode of listening. As we "listen" with all our senses, we become aware of our own feelings—our sadness, or anger, or fear, or affection, sympathy, or antipathy, in response to the other person. And we may discover that we react to certain kinds of people in specific ways: an aggressive person, a smothering person, a dependent person, even an independent person may evoke strong feelings in us, favorable or otherwise. The psychoanalysts refer to these as counter-transference, a term inferring distortion based on the therapist's previous life experience. Naturally, we must question ourselves generally and specifically and take this possibility into consideration. This requires considerable introspection.

While our emotional responses may offer clues, and may suggest much that is valid about the other person, it is also possible that our biases may distort what we hear. We may be listening in a way that refers to our own "images of the past" and not to the patient. And, if that is the case, our emotional responses, and the inferences we draw, will not be valid.

Frequently, we respond emotionally to matters that involve values. To those people whose values agree with ours, we tend to listen carefully and generously. To those whose values conflict with ours, we tend to let our differences interfere with attentive listening, to a greater or lesser extent, depending on the strength of our convictions and the emotions attached to them.

So, another caution is in order: **though we are used to thinking of values as objective, as ideas they are more closely related to belief than to reason**. They emerge, as do our emotional responses, out of our own past. Needless to say, we must explore our emotional responses to our patient. If our reaction is extreme, whether sympathetic or antipathetic, and if we cannot modify it, we must consider giving up our work with that particular person. Whether we choose to separate ourselves, or whether we choose to make this situation an opportunity for mutual learning with our patient, we are again confronted with the importance of knowing ourselves and accepting the knowledge, however unpleasant that may be.

When we make inferences based on our emotional responses, let us keep in mind that they are tentative. If we test our responses and our judgment against that of a third person, a peer, we can better evaluate them. And we may offer them to the patient as impressions to be taken seriously only when we have confirmed them by other evidence.

These feelings, these responses of ours, are therefore to be respected as guides in our relations with other people, which become especially useful as we come to know ourselves better.

Intuition

Feeling must be distinguished from "intuition," which is an indefinable reaction to another person based on nothing as plausible or identifiable as a "feeling." We are informed correctly or not about the other from a place deep inside ourselves that has no other language than that of the "gut."

The person using his or her intuition comes in time to know it and to trust it as a fine tool, becoming free to use it as an artist uses his or her medium. But intuition borders on the mystical and unknown aspects of our lives. It must, therefore, always be used with humility and balance, and with respect for its fragility. It is a gift that illusions of omnipotence and ambition will destroy.

When our actions involve another life, we must trust our intuition as a guide, always to be carefully validated by concrete evidence.

Looking

When we use our eyes, what does the patient's body language tell us? Do their words match their physical gestures, or are they at odds? Are they saying how "cool" things are and, at the same time, ripping their nails from their fingers— or how open and relaxed they feel, while they twist their body into pretzel shapes?

As we watch, we see some familiar gestures and expressions that we have ready words for: uptight, choked up, two-faced, tight-fisted, starry-eyed, wry, twisted, pained. Do the person's eyes make direct contact or do they seem vacant? Are there tremors, sweating, agitation, or an unreal calm? These physical gestures and attitudes are indicators of underlying feelings and personality.

There have been many attempts to classify or type people. They are understandable attempts to organize our experience and make us more secure in our relationships, diagnosis, and treatment. Sheldon's work earlier in the century[3,3a] the skull measurements of the last century and of the Nazis, ancient Chinese physiognomy and face reading[4] (including Dr. Shen[5] and Dr. Mar[6]), the System of Correspondences, the Enneagram, and recently, the Beinfield/

Korngold[7] system, are examples of such classifications. The *Diagnostic and Statistical Manual of Mental Disorders* (DSM)[8] is perhaps the ultimate attempt to classify mental illness and personality. Each has its merits and each its dangers. When we move from the individual to the general something is lost. I prefer the individual and I am grateful to a medicine that gives me the tools to know each person.

"Looking with the third eye" is the vision counterpart of "listening with the third ear." Observing changes in color, position, and movement as a person communicates with words is more revealing than the words. A patient who was constantly praising the therapist's insights and simultaneously shoving both hands to the side of the chair he was sitting in indicated the opposite. When this behavior was gently pointed out to the patient, the humor of the situation got the better of any resentment and the observation led to a more accurate register of the patient's feelings, which revealed a great deal about his relationship to authority and his ability to undermine it surreptitiously.

Touch (Assessment)

This is the earliest form of contact in human experience, and it evokes the deepest feelings. We can learn so much from a touch, from a handshake. For example—the "too glad" hand, the overpowering grip, the "limp rag," the "sweaty palm"—they are all familiar, and they all bear a message, as do the people who clutch, the people who stroke and stimulate, the people who, in contrast, "stand off" as do the people who "make our hair stand on end" and the others who "bathe us in a warm glow," those who "give us the cold shivers," or those who "put us into a hot sweat." Our skin is, indeed, a valuable sensor of the people and the world around us.

A great deal of information is gleaned from traditional diagnostic techniques that involve sophisticated methods of palpation such as pulse diagnosis and palpation of the abdomen and the channels of acupuncture.

Smell

The development of this sense was the mark of the most accomplished fictional investigators, from Sherlock Holmes to Hercule Poirot! If, as therapists, we ignore the evidence of our noses, we are neglecting an important diagnostic tool. We must not ignore the odor of alcohol, of glue, of marijuana, for these odors are clues to states of mind, to strategies for coping. We should not ignore body odors, for they, too, are clues: poorly nourished people have a certain smell; unwashed bodies have a certain smell. Some amphetamines leave the user with an identifiable unpleasant odor on the breath. And emotions produce odors: the odor of fear is unmistakable, and familiar to us. The odor of suspicion and danger is especially well known among "primitive" people. Within the System of Correspondences in CM, each element is associated with an odor.

Reception and Processing (Thinking)

The link between reception and response is the inner processing of information that we have harvested by listening. This harvest becomes transformed by the use of our mind into usable knowledge. It is, so to speak, changed from the raw product into an edible, digestible food for thought. Thinking organizes our contact with reality, our experience.

We listen intuitively, emotionally, with our senses and our feelings. We pull all of our impressions together with "thinking," or that part of our minds that we associate with reason or logic. As we listen, we wonder how certain things go together: why does this young man, who says that he resents his home, return to it over and over again? Why does this woman talk endlessly about how badly her mother treats her but never mentions her father? Our mind tells us that the balance is off, that things do not add up or make sense. We realize, from what she says, that one person is as she is; that another person is avoiding telling us his whole story. Logic tells us that something is missing.

We begin with an assumption, a premise: birds fly; humans do not. We add another: we are human. We conclude, logically, that we cannot fly. So, logic is one way of approaching a problem, another tool. It, too, must be used cautiously, for it does not necessarily yield truth. Consider, for example, the premise based on general experience that liquids get dense as temperature decreases. It should follow logically that water is denser at $0\,°C$ than at $4\,°C$. But that is not true; water at $0\,°C$ is less dense than at $4\,°C$, as experiment bears out. So, our premise about liquids is not universal, and the generalizations we build on it may not yield the truth.

When we make assumptions or generalizations, not about water but about people, we need to be still more wary. If we begin with the premise that working for money is good and idleness evil, or with the premise that short hair indicates respect for authority and long hair symbolizes rebellion, we may be led to mistaken conclusions. For these premises, though they are widely held, are not universal. To treat them as if they were, to draw inferences from them, will not bring us close to the truth of any individual case. Of course, some of our assumptions are valid. But they are never sacred. They always need to be checked.

Logic is important, primarily because it helps us to raise and formulate questions. It helps us to see when something is out of place; that something may be missing in an otherwise complete picture. It leads us to ask whether the person speaking is telling the truth, or deceiving him- or herself as well as the therapist. These questions that logic leads us to, we must remember, imply judgment; they are aids to understanding.

A cautionary note

Reasoning and logic have their limitations. The practitioner, for example, may overly depend upon reason as a source of security; depend upon reason as a response to chaos. If the patient then creates confusion, the practitioner's anxiety may interfere with his or her focus on the patient. Confusion may be a necessary state of affairs in some circumstances and for some period of time, and the therapist needs to learn to live with it comfortably.

Interaction and Communication

Derogation

It is possible, as we have already noted, for two people to say almost anything to each other, provided they say it in a way that does not "put down" the other person. Derogation, putting down, is an attempt by one person to control another, or to enhance him- or herself by making the other person seem less worthwhile. When the patient greets our caring with repeated skepticism, that is derogation. It is one of the most commonly used weapons in human encounters, a weapon that destroys people and relationships. If you, the practitioner, are tempted to use this weapon, if you sincerely feel you are "better" than your patient, stay out of that therapeutic relationship.

Feedback-specific Methods

These involve **humility, validation,** and **clarification** (including **repetition**), **questioning, reframing, interpretation, insight and perspective**, and **working through**.

Humility

Of the many challenging tasks we are faced with in life, learning what is in another person's mind and heart is perhaps the most difficult. From the outset, we must accept that we know a good deal less than we imagine about almost everything, and especially about another person. Recognizing our inherent limitations to know "the other" is the safest posture we can assume as therapists both for ourselves and for the other person. One must depend on the confluence of many approaches to knowing before acting. Too many in our time believe too strongly in the accuracy of whimsical impulse and too little in the hard work necessary to mine the truth. There is truth in the statement, "Trust (oneself) but verify."

Validate and Clarify the Data

Above all, we must be certain that we have perceived correctly. We must check and re-check our perceptions with the patient, to be certain that we agree on all points and to ascertain that he or she knows that we are listening carefully and getting accurate information.

Repetition is an exact replay of the message we have received. It is a way of ascertaining that we have heard correctly, an important aspect of communication that we discussed earlier in relation to logic and premises. If we hear faultily, we may adopt false premises on which to base our reasoning and our conclusions. Then, everything that follows between practitioner and patient is, to some extent, based on misunderstanding.

Misperceived, incorrect information should be corrected at once, misunderstandings cleared up immediately, for error and misunderstanding will misdirect the line of our inquiry and disrupt our relations with the patient. Information checked and mutually agreed upon is a valuable resource for future reference, especially when stories begin to change.

Clarification can be accomplished when ideas are played back, sometimes as we go along and sometimes by way of summary. As well as using repetition to keep the record straight, we play back in order to establish agreement, and to encourage the sense that this work is a mutual endeavor. Not only does the acupuncturist make sure that he or she understands, but also that the patient knows this. Then, when the matter we have agreed on is raised again in another context, we can return to the original earlier agreement for confirmation and support. Of course, agreement, understanding, and comprehension do not happen all at once.

We should strive for early clarification of certain salient questions. What, in the patient's life, is a problem to him or her at this time? What would he or she like to change? What is his or her motivation to change? If we cannot make sense of what we have heard, or if we repeat it inaccurately, we need clarification; and we should invite it, for the very effort will bring into the open many aspects of the issue that were not immediately obvious. Thus, the work of clarification is sometimes an integral part of the work of change. And it is basic to the art of communication.

Communication between people is an endless series of corrections (of errors of perception or understanding or interpretation). This kind of exchange strengthens and deepens all relationships. It is, in all of life, a never-ending activity. If it can get started in the therapeutic relationship, the process can carry over to other relationships (and will, of course, benefit the therapist as well as the patient).

Naturally, a part of each one of us—not only the patient—wishes to avoid clarification of our problems. In the service of repeated clarification, it is helpful for the acupuncturist to summarize at the end of each session what they think they have heard, so that the patient and the acupuncturist may be sure that they have been listening to the same things. The differences may be more significant than opening new areas to explore.

In the therapeutic situation, therefore, we need to pay attention to the means people use to avoid clarity. One common means of doing so is to avoid definite statements about ourselves. Another is to avoid taking a position, for example, by asking questions that cannot settle the issues they raise (often rhetorical questions): "Oh, why did I ever leave school?" In the therapeutic situation, we convert these evasive questions into statements: "I left school because …" and we leave it to the patient to finish them. If he or she refuses, we do so, by way of demonstration. Of course, our version may be quite wrong. But that, too, has value; it will offer an opportunity for correction by the patient, who, in the process of correcting us, will finally commit him- or herself on the subject about which he of she previously had nothing to say.

At this stage, when our relationship with the patient is growing, it is of great value to them that they make statements. It helps strengthen them from the inside. They take a risk when they make a statement, which they have not taken when they ask a question. Accepting that risk, daring to look inside, they begin to feel responsible for what they see, what they once feared too much to see.

Once we are clear about an issue, it is difficult to avoid the next step: to act. Often the action that follows clarity is fraught with risks that we fear to take, judging them to be threats to our security. Once we act, we are responsible, visibly committed to steps that others may respond negatively to. If, for whatever reason, we feel that we cannot stand on our own, that we cannot live with disapproval, we will avoid, first of all, the clarity that leads to action. Therefore, it is vital that the therapist explores with patients the consequences of acting on their clarity or new insights before they do so.

A patient I was treating with acupuncture had a sudden epiphany one day that one reason he did not like his wife was because she had fat ankles. Before I could stop him he bolted from the room, ran home, and disgorged these feelings to her. She was understandably devastated and equally understandably dissuaded him from continuing to work with me. We never had a chance to process this insight in terms of what it meant about him because he "acted out" rather than contained his new awareness.

Question the Data

Having established that we agree about the data, we are obligated to question it without confrontation. We cannot directly impugn the patient's honesty without destroying the relationship. We can say, "Since so much of your present dilemma is an outcome of these experiences, we certainly want to be absolutely sure that they are exactly as you recall." That leaves the subject open to detailed review that might in some cases involve the opinion of other people's recollections and experiences of the same events.

Most often, the problem with the accuracy of data is less in the specific details of events and more in the interpretations of these events at the time of their occurrence or later. If there is one subject that overshadows the rest in terms of the focus of most psychotherapies, it is this process of delineating the observed from the interpretation.

It has been my experience that the best and sometimes only way this can be untangled is within the framework of the therapeutic relationship. When this is a significant discomforting issue in the person's life that might be identified by the patient as one source of their pain, it is wise to anticipate, with the patient, that this issue is bound to occur during one or many acupuncture sessions, and is "grist for the therapeutic mill."

Over and over again, the observation and the interpretation must be sorted, until the patient begins to initiate the process on his or her own. The incentive is the relief of pain. While it is true that some people only know that they are alive if they feel pain, most would rather live without it and are willing to consider changing entrenched patterns rather than continue to suffer.

In the most serious conditions, the observation of an event is interpreted and distorted even before the event unfolds. Here the person's fear is too great to reconsider the only safety he or she has ever felt. He or she is capable of and willing to endure the inevitable accompanying hurt rather than endure the threat of being involved in changing this seemingly life-preserving system.

However, with patience, even the most entrenched maladaptive system is susceptible to change if keeping it is clearly associated with the pain in a person's life. The openings into a place in the system where the patient has even the smallest doubts or awareness is sometimes enough.

One example is that of a person whose experience of being hurt by others involved not what was said but the inflection of the speaker's voice. She voluntarily acknowledged her sensitivity to sound when the subject was raised, creating the possibility of re-examining the events leading to hurt and alienation. The practitioner could question her interpretation of the inflections of voices without challenging her perceptions, but by exploring the subject of her auditory sensitivity from other areas of experience.

Reframing

Reframing is an essential feedback device, a restatement of the issues with a new viewpoint. This means injection of a new, yet related, idea into a set of already-known related ideas. We play back the new arrangement to the patient in the hope that the new element will illuminate the other, familiar ideas. And that, we hope, will lead to redirection of thought and activity.

People who seek help need this readjustment of perspective, for their focus is narrow and they cannot see how they are "stuck." They cannot see that their attitudes, perceptions, feelings, and behavior have trapped them; they need to find out how they have brought this about. Our restatement is a clarifying device, and it will help them to come "unstuck." It may be that they have focused on what is not a problem, and overlooked what is. It may be that they are driven in two opposing directions. Or, it may be that their expectations are unrealistic. When they understand how they have reached an impasse, they can begin to break through it.

Example

Mr. Smith's original reason for coming to see a psychiatrist was a recent homosexual episode, in which he visited a remote part of a beach and met a man whom he followed into the bushes, where they masturbated each other. Am I a homosexual? This is the fearful question that crosses Mr. Smith's mind and that he would like to have answered.

During this first hour, Mr. Smith said that he had had only one other such experience, occurring some years ago in Denmark while he was on vacation. He met a group of homosexual Americans on the beach. One of them tried to get him to go to his house, but Mr. Smith said he had to catch a train. They met again at the train station, and he finally agreed to accompany this person to his house, where he allowed him to masturbate him. After each of these episodes, he promised himself that it would never happen again and after some tortured hours put the entire experience out of his mind.

Why did it happen again now? He doesn't know. During the first hour, Mr. Smith describes himself as a lonely, almost "alone" man, who is unable to bring himself to do the creative work that he feels is in him. He is a journalist who works for a well-known magazine. He collects all the information, writes the story, and then it appears under someone else's name with whatever slant this person decides to use—frequently being considerably different from what he would have said, which often has embarrassing repercussions. He is a Democrat working for a Republican magazine. He has always wanted to write a novel, but he has never been able to do it, start on it, or even have an idea. He has been obsessed with saving enough money at his present job to take off a few years for a creative effort.

He has no close friends; lives alone; has never had intercourse with a woman, despite his age and several opportunities; has no hobbies or interests; and does little for entertainment. He has a girlfriend with whom he does everything except have full intercourse.

My first reframing conveyed to Mr. Smith was that while his presenting problem was deciding his sexuality, it was the emptiness of his life that conveyed the deepest and most lasting dilemma. The endless questioning of his sexuality put off his awareness that there was no real relationship in his life, male or female, or even with himself in terms of creativity. The rooms of his "house" were empty of others and also of himself.

His homosexuality might be considered as a tentative and tenuous attempt to bridge the gap to others. It would seem that, for the time being, the attraction of these excursions lay in their excitement, this being the only activity in his life that aroused and stimulated him, the only one that made him feel safely alive. He seemed to have had many obsessional ways of keeping his emotional emptiness out of awareness, especially by the dilemma of deciding his sexuality.

Mr. Smith was struck by this way of looking at his life and seemed somewhat incredulous, but immensely absorbed by what he was hearing. He was transferred to a long-term assignment in Africa by his employer and we continued our conversation by letter for about two years during which this reframing was the principal subject.

We see, then, that when the issues are clarified through reframing, the therapist and patient are in a position to agree on the "real" problems they are to work on together. These "real" problems are rarely the ones presented at first contact. "Real" problems are usually self-resolving. "Unreal" problems are endlessly repeated in a vicious cycle that leads back to itself with no resolution.

Interpretation

Once the "real" problem has been identified, the next step in the process of change is the practitioner's attempt to tie its many threads into a recognizable and workable life-fabric: to offer an explanation. We call this "interpretation." If the patient is ensnared in an emotional or mental mire as Mr. Smith was, interpretation is one necessary ingredient in loosening the fixed patterns of misery. What were the causes in Mr. Smith's early life that forced him to choose the safety of living in a dispassionate rather than passionate way? While interpretation by itself, without the working through (repeating the process of interpretation and reframing until the patient has a breakthrough in understanding), is not sufficient for change to occur, it is an important ingredient in the process.

Example

In an example involving both reframing and interpretation, a young man found, after a number of years of living with a young woman, that she had withdrawn from him almost completely. He lived his life in fantasy. When, for various reasons, his fantasy life broke down, he was faced with the barrenness of his real life. He experienced only total rejection and enormous anger at his girlfriend.

Then he began to see things from another viewpoint. For reasons stemming from early childhood, illuminated by interpretation, he defended himself against hurt by never needing, only filling others' needs (unless the need was for him). In his relationship with his girlfriend, she slowly found herself unneeded.

Being needed by the person one loves gives one the opportunity to give and express that love. He would give her no chance to care for him, would need nothing, and demand nothing. So, she replaced him—with a thoroughbred horse who "thoroughly" needed her full time and attention. Once the therapist helped him achieve a new outlook on his life (reframing), and see the subtle way he first rejected others before they rejected him, the possibilities for growth in his life appeared. The perceptual screen cleared, and the information reaching him more closely approximated reality.

Perception is the monitor through which the world passes from our senses to our response. The accuracy of our response to the world depends, to a large degree, on how little our screen distorts reality. Our problem is that a defective screen may be rigid and the messages we get consistently inaccurate. The result is a developing pattern of maladaptations. We do not know that there may be another way of experiencing the message coming from the outside world until we share our experiences with another person who encourages us to try new lenses in our perceptual screen.

Insight and Perspective

As the process of integrating material and of interpreting and interpolating it goes on, as it is repeated over and over, it leads both the therapist and the patient to the greater awareness that we call "insight." We mean by this a depth and breadth of understanding of ourselves and of others, which is akin to a growing wisdom. For example, the woman discussed above with the extreme auditory sensitivity and misperceptions of voice inflections needed to realize ultimately that the negative messages being received could be reflections of her own self-image. This realization is called insight.

In the service of developing insight, we attempt to use repetitious feedback to broaden the range of our perceptions, to generalize. If, in discussing a specific incident, we learn something about the patient, we try to relate it to other specific incidents, so that it may contribute to our general understanding of his or her personality. We move, thus, from the specific to the general and from the particular situation to the whole person—the ultimate source of both the problem and its solution.

We live by our own point of view. We act according to our perspective. We may fail repeatedly in our efforts to fashion life according to that picture. The view of ourself and our situation from a new perspective creates an opening in any life impasse. All of the techniques discussed above—repetition, clarification, reframing, and interpretation, and the resulting insight—serve this end.

Working Through

Repetition, clarification, reframing, interpretation, and insight sharpen focus, stimulate movement, and redirect energy. Flow and movement are vital to the therapeutic relationship, as they are to life; without this constant unceasing passage it stagnates and dies. These techniques encourage the patient's increasingly accurate perception of him- or herself and the world.

This repetitive process is known as "working through." It qualifies as work in the most rigorous meaning of that word. Indeed, all the contact we have described is essentially hard work, inspired though it may be at times.

Awareness

All of the devices discussed are in the service of advancing "awareness." Being completely in the moment is the fulfillment of being.

Instructions (Essential Qualities)

The Patient's Dilemma

The patient generally comes heavily burdened by repeated failure to establish successful relations with other people, to achieve satisfaction and the self-esteem and sense of security that are essential to self-fulfillment.

What are these satisfactions? They have been summed up as being and becoming as much ourselves as possible in the constructive context of others doing the same. Usually this involves love and work, a capacity for intimacy, authentic, direct contact across the physical, emotional, and verbal spectrum, from tender touch to appropriate assertion. It means a talent for structure, logic, and organization, along with the ability to function in and tolerate anarchy. Being and becoming suggest respect and self-respect, commitment and responsibility, imagination and creation, values, ethics, and principles. They encompass faith, trust, and the spirit. They include tolerance for the imperfection of all of the above in oneself and in others. All of this is inherent in the expression "satisfaction." A better word is "fulfillment."

Obviously, pursuing these mostly unfulfilled needs means to struggle for them again and again, endlessly, for as long as one lives. Struggling and failing, failing repeatedly, the individual's inherent talents engage in a lifelong attempt at restoration, to set things right. But, since one might have little or no experience in using these inherent talents to make positive contact, and since, indeed, that lack is the source of repeated failure, each successive attempt proves abortive and deepens the inevitable despair. And these efforts have an unforeseen result.

Whenever the path to fulfillment is blocked, the energy turns to impotent rage. Out of this impotence springs hate, vengeance, envy, jealousy, violence, or its alternatives, depression, and finally physical illness. Any one or all of these conditions turns people against others and, inevitably, turns them against themselves. Thus it is that they are caught in a pattern of abuse unless some corrective experience intervenes, some guidance, divine or human.

What is a "pattern of abuse"? A pattern describes something that repeats itself consistently and predictably. In human terms, it is a perception of life that is self-fulfilling. A person is what they feel. If the feeling is hate, then they feel hateful and behave this way, and are hateful.

Example

One woman I knew was enormously jealous of her sister, who she correctly felt was their mother's favorite. She was a prisoner of these feelings. They made her feel ugly and isolated. She could not understand where these feelings about herself came from, so she believed that others thought her ugly and avoided her. This fed her hatred and increased her withdrawal. Her misery began to shape her expression, and a potentially pretty face became vacant; people did in reality begin to avoid her. At the heart of her unhappiness was a longing for the love that her mother could not give. The abuse, as this case illustrates, is the transformation of a healthy need into a poisoned quest.

Given past experience, we can understand that when the patient comes to us they are of two minds. One wishes to reach out, to make contact. At the same time, repeated failures have made a direct approach seem dangerous, perhaps impossible. They may want us near but not too near, for they are frightened. They search for a way to hold us and, at the same time, to keep us away. Their struggle to act on these opposing impulses is painful to them and to us.

For, as they fail to reconcile these opposites, to the extent that their "hang ups" interfere with their impulse to trust us, this reaching out may show itself in twisted, deeply unattractive ways: in silence, in insolence, in a teasing approach and sudden withdrawal, in manipulative games, in provocation, in rejection. All of these maneuvers fashioned their contact in childhood with primary and secondary caretakers who were unavailable in more nourishing ways. Pain in its many forms is preferable to the interpersonal void.

An example of this is the person who is never on time, often to the great inconvenience of other people. This becomes an obvious issue in therapy. What does it mean? While on the surface it may seem to mean many things, at the root it is, however maladaptive, a way of establishing a powerful contact. The medium of that contact is the respondent's frustration and resentment.

In one case it meant that the patient thought herself special, that the rules did not apply to her. For another habitually late patient it meant a profound indecisiveness, an appeal to someone else to take responsibility. For yet another it was a defiant announcement that the practitioner should not take the patient's need for him for granted. Independent of the precise nature of the behavior and its source, the core issue is that each is a method of creating a dependable, albeit unpleasant, form of contact.

While we cannot always depend for essential human contact upon people loving us just for who we are, we can depend upon their anger when they are provoked. A subtle example is the woman who constantly challenged the practitioner's remarks, implying that he lied. Of course, this was infuriating to him. Nevertheless, he came to see these barbs as a form of contact; rousing his anger was the safest way this patient dared devise. And while his anger showed that he cared about her, as his implacability would not, this anger had to be reframed in the context of her peculiar need to make contact in this maladaptive fashion.

Again, these maneuvers, these games of acceptance and rejection, are not to be taken at face value, but to be seen in the light of the patient's fear of a nourishing intimacy.

Acceptance and Positive Experience

Of course, in normal everyday life, people do not put up with this sort of irritation for very long; they tire and withdraw or punish. We therapists must not take this position. Our concern is with helping people develop a mode of life that is comfortably congruent with their needs and reasonably tolerant for those around them. Our effort is to help them recognize their problems and work them through, so that they can function in society. Our interest is rehabilitative, never punitive. Especially in the first stages of a therapeutic relationship, this means accepting patients at the level at which they accept or reject themselves. It is within the framework of their perception of reality that we begin to work, however antithetical their perceptions may be to our own.

When our clients behave in irritating ways we can assume that their past experience with people has been unfortunate. It is important, therefore, that our relations with them are positive. We may at some point want to offer some criticism; we should not offer it until we have established a basis of trust that will allow them to accept it, to see it as helpful.

Above all, we do this by sharply delineating positive talents for living from the destructive ways these talents are employed in the service of maintaining life-giving contact. Positive experience with us (or with others), however small, will in time offset the negative experiences that have been blocking the patient's growth. Even as they continue to seesaw, to play games of acceptance and rejection, we can be reasonably certain the shared experience is constructive. And, as previously mentioned, even if the therapeutic link is interrupted, gains of this kind will not be lost.

Example ───────────────────────────────────────

An example of this seesawing is a young man who ended each session with the words, "I guess we didn't accomplish anything, after all." He felt impelled to undo, to diminish with these words, the meaningful contact we had made together. Why? Because, as much as he needed the contact, he also feared it; he needed distance from it. In a situation of this kind, it is vital that we recognize the patient's internal struggle. That he feels the need for contact is apparent, for he keeps coming back.

───────────────────────────────────────

We tolerate his way of coping, however negative and frustrating. We appreciate his talent for living while endeavoring to separate it clearly from the corruption of that talent in the service of survival under unfavorable circumstances. Why, we might ask, does someone who needs us keep us at a distance?

Example ───────────────────────────────────────

A young man I knew needed emotional and financial support from both of his parents. He was always invited by both of them to indulge his needs. However, there was a price exacted for the indulgence. His father required him to listen for hours on end about his grievances against his mother and the world; and his mother demanded complete subservience to her needs of the moment, even to the extreme of quenching her sexual thirsts. It was extremely difficult for this young man to allow himself, at any level, the awareness of the smallest need for others because that might lead him again to be used as an object rather than loved as an individual.

───────────────────────────────────────

Whatever the specific reason for this keeping of distance, it makes our exchange with the patient difficult, for he or she places little trust in our good intentions and our efforts. This is the heart, the essence of our work. Our task is to expose this lack of trust through insight and change it through new experience. On our side is the life force, the drive for health and fulfillment. Working against us is the terror of change and of the unknown, the belief that one who dares to trust will be undone. And the moment comes when the patient begins to lose this fear; in time a pattern of mutual trust and respect will develop.

Thus, whatever a patient's overt negative behavior, however distasteful its form, we need to recognize its positive intent; however veiled, it is a cry for help, a desperate cry for life. It is vital that we understand it as that, and that we respond adequately, for our work as practitioners is predicated on the principle that human life and growth are grounded in human contact. The creation and continuance of that contact is our primary concern, the ground from which we work. It takes precedence over all other considerations, except where our survival or the survival of other innocent people is at issue. (I expand on this topic in the section on "Objectivity" in Chapter 1, p. 15, and in the section on "Timing" below [p. 68].)

Attention

It is clear that in order "to be" one has to be "seen." For example, the young girl whose father does not see her beauty and charm does not see herself that way either. If he does not touch her in a loving fashion she cannot feel lovable. A young boy who is not heard by his father will never easily gain his full voice in the world. Each child and, ultimately, the adult, is dependent on the quality and quantity of notice he or she receives from each parent and parent surrogates for all developmental needs including to be seen, heard, touched, and responded to, for containment and discipline, in order to "be" all each person can. Fortunately we are capable of repair through healing "contact," over the course of a life even after the malleable era of childhood. With that therapeutic contact comes the healing power of awareness (see above).

Empathy

Empathy (feeling with) is the capacity to sense in oneself accurately another person's feelings, although they are not directly communicated with words. It is akin to tuning in, to finding and resonating with another person's wavelength or perhaps cosmic vibrations. It is fundamental to intimacy and human growth.

Example ———————————————————————————————

Years ago a frightened man came and expressed his grief at finding himself in middle age stuck since childhood in work that suffocated him and denied him the life he felt inside had never been realized. He told a story of endless fear. He was a milliner whose family had immigrated when he was a child, in great poverty as refugees from persecution and certain death. His father was also a milliner and he was apprenticed in this trade as a very young child in order to help the family survive. His father died early and he was left with his mother and siblings and ultimately his own family to support. He had reached the point of despair that needed a voice, and I was moved by that genuine voice.

At some point in the initial interview, this man, who was on the verge of self-destruction, saw tears in my eyes. Later he wrote that at the moment he saw those tears he began to feel a stirring of hope, to feel alive. Unexplainably his fear fell away and he was free. He wrote this to me about a year after I saw him. I was astounded and have never forgot him.

———————————————————————————————

Intuition

Intuition is both a "what" and "how" of the therapeutic relationship and is discussed in both the "Technique of Contact" and "Instructions" sections of this chapter. Like empathy it is fundamental to intimacy and human growth.

If empathy is the sixth sense, intuition is the seventh. The person using intuition over time comes to know it and to trust it as a fine instrument, becoming free to use it as an artist uses a familiar medium. But intuition borders on the mystical and unknown aspects of our lives. It must, therefore, always be used with humility and balance, and with respect for its fragility. It is a gift of possibilities, which illusions of omnipotence and ambition will destroy. It is valuable additional information, never dogma.

Intuition is a valuable dimension of knowing that is sometimes alluded to as a "hunch." Like any other talent, it is stronger in some people than in others. Intuition is related to the little-understood phenomenon of empathy. As explored above, empathy is the capacity to sense in oneself another person's most profound feelings that goes deeper than anything his or her words could convey on paper. Intuition includes much more than just empathy with the person's feelings. It may inform us about his or her entire being, or just important aspects that concern us at any one moment.

Some people fear their intuition. They experience but do not trust the experience and therefore hesitate to act. In today's skeptical world, relying on insight for which we cannot provide scientific, objective evidence is largely unacceptable. It is incumbent upon us to resolve our dilemma with that aspect of knowing and at the same time use it in the context of validation with all the other available diagnostic tools. We must consider it a personal insight perhaps more meaningful about ourselves than the "other" until we can concretely make that connection to the other. Nevertheless, intuition is one of our most valuable resources. Drawing as it does upon all of our previous experience and knowledge, intuition may provide the critical connection and direction in the development of an idea.

Caring

The human animal is a social animal. We need others to encourage us, to help us to clarify our position, to measure ourself and our growth. We reach our highest achievements as participating members of society.

In the therapeutic situation, our care for our patients, and our interest in matters of concern to them (however small, and whether or not we share their views of themselves), create a social bond. That our genuine care is integral to the ongoing therapeutic process and deepens with it, becomes apparent to even an uninvolved, otherwise indifferent patient. Our caring, demonstrated through words and action, creates an indispensable bond.

In every therapeutic relationship, it is essential that we observe the basic premise: to maintain contact, to get in touch, and to keep in touch with the other person. It often requires that we meet some considerable challenges, that we take some risks, that we make sacrifices. But, as long as we maintain contact, we can hope to achieve understanding and change. To the patient, the very effort we expend to maintain contact is a measure of our concern. Even the most withdrawn and reluctant person is touched, moved to a new sense of the situation when they see the trouble we are willing to take to reach them and stay with them.

Furthermore, the practitioner may be the first person for whom the patient returns this caring. It is precious, and we accept it and nourish it. For, as they extend this concern for us, as it covers an increasingly broad spectrum, the patient will grow. Many practitioners are unable to shake off their formal instruction that all of the activities of their patients are only attempts at manipulation. This is a view that derogates the healthy instincts of their patients and puts to rest the real possibility of helping them achieve healthy self-esteem, the lack of which initiated the quest for help in the first place.

Touch (Therapeutic)

Within the first five years of my psychoanalytic training it was increasingly clear to me that touch was the key ingredient missing from the otherwise overly intellectual exercise of psychoanalysis. This awareness had several roots.

In my own therapy, my life was completely changed when a 76-year-old woman arose from her chair and walked across the room to place her hand on my chest. A lifetime of physical and emotional guardedness evaporated in a convulsion of my entire body and being, and though by no means exorcised of all my demons, the aspect leading me down the road to serious mental disability was eliminated. I was in medical college at the time.

The second series of experiences involved the animals who were my constant companions during the years after 1961. I entered the William A. White Institute of Psychiatry and Psychoanalysis in New York in 1955 and began to practice actively following my psychiatric residency in 1956, though I had been "moonlighting" in evening private clinics since 1953. In 1960, I inherited two very high-bred Persian cats from the followers of the recently deceased director of the institute that I was attending.

Beginning in 1961, among my professional associates I include my dog, a Chesapeake Bay Retriever, who was my companion when I worked with adults and children. She could differentiate between those truly in grief and those with "crocodile tears," and would climb on the chest of those in genuine grief.

She made physical contact with those who could not relate to me, many of them schizophrenics, and reinforced what I already felt was missing in psychoanalysis: touch. Physical touch I realized was more necessary to healing than the limiting intellectual exercise characteristic of psychoanalysis.

At the same time, as mentioned above, I was living and working with two cats Mochca and Muki. Muki was a male and extremely friendly to one and all. Mochca, on the other hand, was a killer, approachable only when she was in heat. She could not be touched without coming away with a bloody stump formerly called a hand. However, when the most seriously ill of all my patients, a woman in and out of mental hospitals, sat on my couch, Mochca came out of her hiding place and quietly jumped on her lap, allowing her to pet her freely without any consequences except loud purring. Ultimately this woman took Mochca to live with her, good riddance from my perspective, and Mochca lived to the ripe old age of 23 years. However, more amazing was this woman's remarkable recovery after 15 years of hospitalizations, to marry a wealthy man, have a child, and live "happily ever after" with Mochca to whom we both attributed a significant part of her miraculous recovery.

From my own experience with touch, from a deep sense of the need for it, and these experiences with my animal colleagues, I began my search for methodologies involving touch, and eventually found Ida Rolf's Rolfing,[9] Fritz Perls's gestalt therapy,[10] Alexander Lowen's[11] and John Pierokos's[12] bioenergetics (1967–75) and found all these forms of touch a physical assault on the body, based on the concept of overcoming "defenses" and "resistance" in the physical as well as mental bodies. I had previously read Wilhelm Reich's *Character Analysis*[13] in the psychoanalytic institute.

It was pure serendipity when I stepped into Dr. Van Buren's office in England in 1971 and found myself absolutely certain that I had found, without knowing anything about it, the medicine (CM) that I had always meant when I said at the age of 2½ that I wanted to be a doctor. Here was touch in a medical setting that was synchronic with my concept of nourishing the soul and body rather than attacking it (as is the case with bioenergetics and Rolfing).

Others have written about touch in the context of healing. Dr. David Bresler,[14] Director of the Pain Control Unit at UCLA tells his patients "to use hugging as a part of their treatment for pain" with great success. Dr. Harold Voth, Senior Psychiatrist at the Menninger Foundation states that "hugging is an excellent tonic" and "hugging can lift depression, enabling the body's immune system to become tuned up. Hugging breathes fresh life into a tired body and makes you feel younger and more vibrant. In the home, daily hugging will improve relationships and significantly reduce friction." He also said, "The warm meaningful embrace can have a very positive effect on people, particularly during times of widespread stress and tension like today."[15]

Dr. Robert Rynearson, who is Chairman of the Psychiatry Department at Scott and White Clinic in Temple, Texas, says, "I'm convinced that the tender embrace can prevent or cure a host of different problems," and "A hug can have an astonishing therapeutic effect by providing a sense of companionship and happiness." "Researchers discovered that when a person is touched, the amount of hemoglobin in their blood increases significantly," said Helen Colton, author of *The Gift of Touch*[16] and "my 15 years of research have convinced me that regular hugging can actually prolong life by curing harmful depression and stimulating a stronger will to live." Pamela McCoy, RN, who trains nurses at Grant Hospital in Columbus, Ohio said, "We found that people who are hugged or touched can often stop medication and go to sleep."

There are of course, dangers associated with touch in a therapeutic relationship, especially between a male practitioner and a female patient. It is a challenge to maintain the boundaries between the healing power of touch and the sexual attraction that such healing power can engender. This does not imply simply a question of predatory impulses on the part of the therapist but also from the sexual impulses that touch may arouse in the patient.

Sympathy and Support

These are two attitudes, two reactions to other people that have been misunderstood in recent years; they have had a "bad press." They have been confused with "coddling," "spoiling," and "pity," and associated with weakness in both the giver and the receiver. Mistaken in the giver for their presumed susceptibility to manipulations, and for a spurious sense of superiority they are presumed to derive from their charitable act; in the receiver for their admission of need (which is taken to be self-demeaning).

But sympathy and support are never to be thought shameful. They are the offspring of empathy, an essential emotion, the very basis of our connection with one another. It is the heart of all understanding, and understanding is the goal of all communication. Without understanding we are isolated. We are afraid. We may die.

Too much of any good thing may hurt and weaken us. But too little is worse. Sympathy and support should be given freely, openly, intelligently (that is, with measure, with a sense of how much is too much, how little too little), and with appropriate timing. We learn to judge appropriateness by trial and error, making mistakes and correcting them. If we withhold support or sympathy for fear of being criticized as "too easy," we will have denied an ingredient indispensable to growth.

Flexibility

Flexibility is the essence of health, the goal of all growth experience. When we are compelled rigidly to follow only one way we become sick. We are well when we are inwardly free to make a choice. While rigidity dooms us to function in very limited circumstances, flexibility allows us to adjust to many different situations without compromising our principles. Harry Stack Sullivan[17] defined neurosis as an immutable rigidly unchanging pattern of perception and response. Some place this in the context of the forward movement of normal developing maturity, from dependence on parenting figures to responsibility and the assumption of the parenting role. Those who do not pass through this "rite of passage" are doomed to be children forever.

Hope

Hope is the energy that drives life through stress and obstacles. Hope is engendered when a new perspective shows the way beyond an old impasse or out of a vicious cycle of misery, in the context of all that we have referred to as "respect." Hope is engendered when the practitioner asks "What is the 'good' in all this 'bad'?" "Where is the 'talent' within the destructive life patterns?"

Example

A young unmarried woman with three children came to see me for reasons I cannot remember. She had successfully raised these children by illegally milking government agencies of money and services that she was not entitled to. While she had done this successfully for years, she spent all of her time and energy ingeniously manipulating the system, always one step ahead of the law and in a constant state of tension and anxiety.

There seemed no solution to her anxiety except to draw her attention to her peculiar talent to bend the rules brilliantly, and endlessly outfox every level of government and the laws of the land with nothing to show for it except a paltry few hundred dollars a month. I pointed out that people with a fraction of her talent made fortunes doing the same thing legally as lawyers, and perhaps it was now time to reconsider her options. One of these was to get the government to send her to back to school for vocational rehabilitation with the ultimate goal of becoming a lawyer. As I recall she had some college credits.

She followed this advice, and when we were last in contact a few years after these discussions she was a lawyer and doing well. Hope came first when she realized her talent, and then increased with the realization of its more favorable employment. Hope was inherent in the practitioner's focus on the "positive" as a way out of the obvious "destructiveness" that imprisoned her, a destructiveness that could only grow with harsh judgment and no way out.

Timing

There are two aspects to timing. The first concerns the timing of the patient and second concerns the timing of the practitioner.

With regard to the patient, what brings the patient to seek help at this particular moment in his or her life? As a general rule, with apologies to the exceptions, people seek help to be able to continue a destructive lifestyle without having to pay the penalty: ill health.

People seek help from a health practitioner because they suffer from a symptom and the practitioner's part of the therapeutic contract is to identify a medical condition that explains that symptom. For example, it is relatively easy for an acupuncturist to identify the condition in CM terms, and there are endless acupuncture and herbal protocols to treat CM conditions. However, it is the obligation of the practitioner to go beyond the symptom and the condition and encourage the patient to search his or her lifestyle for the root cause, including the lifestyle of his or her parents before, during, and after the pregnancy with the patient.

The time the patient chooses to seek help is the time when his or her life system is breaking down and it is important for the practitioner not to allow the stress that created the problem to continue by ameliorating the symptom, except in perhaps in debilitating conditions or life-threatening emergencies. And even here, the intervention should include the proviso that the root issue is still fair game once the urgent situation is resolved.

Therefore, the patient's timing is a function of the stress of their life and the terrain on which the stress is manifesting that brings them to the health care provider. The practitioner reads this equation to the best of his or her ability. However, the "iron" of this person's life is in the "fire" and it is the practitioner's timing to "strike at the iron while it is still hot." The timing of this contact between patient and practitioner can be life-saving. Our task is to help patients see that what they are doing will not work, that it will never work. Only when they realize this will they want to do something different.

How do we tell patients something they do not wish to hear without alienating them? The timing of our remarks depends to some extent on the strength and flexibility of the contact we have established. In this, their expressions and body language can guide us, sometimes better than their words.

However, in the context of the practice of CM, that contact is probably of relatively recent origin and the average length of the therapeutic contract relatively short. So CM practitioners must act swiftly as well as decisively. I do not tell patients "I *think* the marijuana is destroying your liver and leaving you paralyzed to realize and to follow through on your best intentions." I tell them that "the examination, the pulse, the tongue and their words (even blood chemistries and biomedical imaging), inform us that a drug is destroying your liver and your life." Objectivity, free of personal opinion, is the key to rendering a listener open to a message that he or she would otherwise resist. It is easy to resist people; it is hard to oppose a pulse or a tongue that have no personal agenda. The practitioner's persona disappears in favor of the data. A lifetime of clinical practice taught me the truth of this approach. Within that framework almost anything can be said directly as long as one says it without derogation and intimidation.

During my residency, disturbed people were brought to the Admitting Office of Bellevue Psychiatric Hospital by their families, friends, and the police, for incarceration, resisting and denying the seriousness of their condition. However, alone with the doctor they almost invariably continued their struggle until the doctor dispassionately said, "Look. Let us leave everyone else out of this—your spouse, your family, and/or the police. Make believe they do not exist. Both you and I know that you are too terrified, too scared to be anywhere except just where you are now." And, in my memory, none of the hundreds of people who were confronted this way ever disagreed or continued to resist hospitalization by me or my colleagues who practiced the same approach.

Acceptance (Won't and Can't)

Let us begin with the initial meeting. When they first come to health practitioners, patients have some notion that their life—"things"—could be different. Indeed, they have been toying with this notion for some time. Other people have urged them to change, have expected them to, have reproached them, have threatened them, and have accused them of not wanting to change. Worse, people have thrown it in their face: that it is only because they stubbornly refuse to change that they continue to be troubled (with whatever it is that disrupts their life). And change, they are led to believe, is simply a matter of willpower.

Some "bad habits," it is true, can be reversed by simply retraining. But in many life situations, it is not true; we are not able to change simply by exercising willpower. And this is always the case when the feelings that motivate our behavior are out of the reach of our understanding. Then our actions take us somehow, we do not know how, far from our intentions, which is to say that we are unaware of ourselves. It may be that we are too frightened to know ourselves, so we block our perceptions. That does not mean that we do not want to change, but that until we overcome our fright and our maladaptive self-protective behavior we will not be in a position to change. Until then, hamstrung as we are, we may simply be trying ways that do not work. In such a situation, we must assume that, to a reasonable degree, we want to change but can't.

Do we accept the premise that we cannot do some things by ourselves and for ourselves? Yes. The therapeutic relationship is based on the assumption that one person sometimes needs another in order to change "I can't" into "I can." It is, essentially, a somewhat formalized extension of the life process: all people need others; the people we work with need others to an unusual degree. Their needs are not different in kind from anyone else's needs.

Example

A young woman came to see me and talked about her past life in a monotonous monologue for over an hour. When she finished, I asked in a friendly way why she chose to bore me for an hour, when we both knew she was on the verge of suicide. Thus, I conveyed to her my acute awareness of her underlying despair and desperation, which she conveyed to me through her "deadening" recitation. Coming from a finishing school background, she was "bucking up" in public while quietly slipping into madness and despair. No one seemed to recognize her desperation. Previous practitioners had analyzed the details of her boring "rap" instead of recognizing the boring aspect of the "rap" as a camouflaged way of saying, "If you feel the deadliness of this, you will know how close to death I am."

When I recognized, acknowledged, and focused on the real message, she became able to express her despair, to let go of her pretenses, to engage in a therapeutic relationship that did not require that she appear "perfect." The crux of the problem, she now began to see, was the false image, with its false expectations, that had shielded her from the "reality" of herself. The point is that it took another person's recognition of the facade, and the desperation it hid, for change to become possible. She could not do this for herself.

It is a fallacy to expect patients to function in the therapeutic relationship in a manner other than that for which they were seeking help. For a patient coming late, or being unable to communicate is not "resistance," it is their life adaptation in order to survive, often since the beginning of their life. I had a patient who was always interrupting, who later explained his very disturbing habit as the only way he could get attention for his needs as a child in his family.

Dependence, Independence, and Initiative

Continuing our discussion of "can't" and "won't," who can deny that ultimately each person is responsible for him- or herself? Independence is an inherent ingredient of life's drive to "become." However, balanced and rational dependency is the modus vivendi of "becoming." Just as a child depends upon a mature person to be able to develop, a crippled person needs a crutch until he or she can heal and walk. For change to occur in the areas of "cannot," one human being needs the dependable collaboration of another. The hurtful behavior, attitudes, habits of mind that arose out of bad experience with people can be corrected only by a new and good experience with people, often with the practitioner.

In the therapeutic situation, we have a foundation for the movement towards self-sufficiency in the patient's very act of seeking help. This is a responsible and independent act. It is the evidence of this basic drive to "become," which the treatment builds upon to help realize independence within the context of responsibility to others.

At the different stages of growth toward a balanced self-sufficiency, some degree of leaning and dependency is necessary, especially during transitions. The trick is to let people lean so that they can grow stronger (not weaker). They must lean to grow and we must deal with our own aversion to dependency, if we have one.

There are those patients for whom lacking initiative is a principal problem in their life. As CM practitioners, we are called upon to deal with problems involving decision-making and the ability to move forward or retreat appropriately (liver *yang* [gallbladder]). Often people come to us who cannot execute their ideas into appropriate action (pericardium *yang* [triple burner]). These conditions are extremely common in our time as the result of the use of "cold" "substances of abuse" such as marijuana, LSD, heroin. While the correct needles and herbs can make a significant difference, the CM practitioner is also called upon to become involved in a human relationship, as illustrated by the following examples.

Personally, I am not fearful of a dependency that I see as a necessity in the course of individuation, a dependency that failed to lead to growth and maturity during the appropriate stage of development and must be revisited within a therapeutic relationship. At the same time that I assume an active role in the areas of true dependency, patients are encouraged to assume an active role in the areas where they are capable of responsibility. Thus, we have a healing alliance. I become that part of their ego that is missing in order for them to move ahead with what they can do, and from that they learn by example while the CM intervention strengthens them so they can assume that role themselves.

Example

The following example illustrates this alliance. A 38-year-old man was referred to me for herbal therapy saying that he had been smoking marijuana since aged 14 and "shooting" heroin for the last 9 years. He slept all day and stayed up all night watching television in order to forget the guilt he felt for sleeping all day while avoiding the work to which he had committed himself and which he was capable of doing well. He did not want to be gainfully promoting a society with which he strongly disagreed and was escaping the struggle that was inevitable in fighting for the things he believed and against those with which he disagreed. He had never been strong enough for that battle.

Yet, he said that he wanted to be healthy and knew that to accomplish this the drugs had to go, and that he had to function, that he needed supervision and direction to accomplish this. This direction began by listing all of his work projects and their priorities as well as those that could be done outside on rain-free days and inside when it rained (he was a carpenter).

However, he could not awake in the morning to begin work. Since I am an early riser we agreed that I would call him every day at 7:00 a.m. and review the day's work. We also reviewed the previous day. For the first time in years he worked during the day and slept at night and became drug-free with a brief exception. I have worked with many others like him for long periods with meaningful success.

Many of the people CM practitioners will see are those whose adaptations for survival are less acceptable either to society or to themselves. The young man we discussed above escaped into drugs in order to live with that part of himself that would have been intolerable to his ego: his fear of fighting for what he believed. Looking in the mirror of his own mind and of the society in which he lived, he saw the word "coward," and being unable to tolerate that condemnation, he escaped through mind-numbing substances, leading to a living or ultimate death. To break out of this destructive cycle, he needed to lean on the strengths of the practitioner until he could develop his own.

Here we face one of the hardest lessons of all: that learning of any kind (standing, walking, and so on) requires thousands of trials and errors before it becomes that other kind of learning: trial and success. Many of us give up after the first defeat. For this reason especially, the patient needs our support and guidance. We must, therefore, be always ready to accept real dependency, to solve immediate problems beyond the operant level of competency of the patient, to assist them as they grow in independence, to share decision-making, to rejoice with them along the way, and to support them when necessary, to keep our goals in sight and—perhaps paramount—to keep constant vigilance over ourselves so that we too may grow and avoid feelings of superiority that can only be destructive to any interpersonal relationship.

We have already said that maladaptive behavior develops in a particular early life setting as the only childhood behavior that meets the need to stay in contact while staying intact, to survive. Some of these survival techniques are ego-syntonic (acceptable to the aims of the ego) and are acceptable, even encouraged in society. The "successful" driven person who is unable to love and neglects family and friends while accumulating power, wealth, and recognition is well known to us as the "type A personality" generally brought to therapy by a physical consequence of their emptiness such as a heart attack.

Drug abuse is a special and extreme example for acupuncturists in which the issue of dependence is primary. For abusers—people who use drugs to their own detriment—have learned to substitute drug-induced experience for human experience, often because they have found drugs more dependable than people (more dependable, too, than themselves). To satisfy any given need, whether for excitement or for peace, for sensuality, for perception, for insight, or just for relief of pain—they depend on drugs. Thus, drugs replace human contact.

The difficult task of a therapeutic relationship is to reverse that tendency. Our emphasis must be on people and not on drugs, not on pills. It must be on the positive talent that people bring even to maladaptive behavior, not the behavior. Otherwise, as with drug dependency, if we fail to focus on the patient, we risk entanglement in the obsessive scheme of things, in games of drug-talk, displays of drug know-how and recitations of drug experiences. All this we will discover, are devices to avoid human contact and to stave off the threat of rejection.

Example

A young man, aged 17, had been abandoned by his mother when he was about 14 years old. He stayed with his father, who arranged their space as if they were roommates sharing an apartment. They led separate lives, each bringing home a woman of his choice to share his bed. The father, a very successful businessperson, generally ate away from home, and the boy fended for himself. He quickly became involved with drugs, especially with amphetamines. By the time I saw him he was becoming extremely paranoid. He was hospitalized, became violent, and was required to have male nurses around the clock. Because of the amphetamines, he could not sleep. By chance, the male nurses were all black men who were mature and had seen a great deal of life. They were intelligent, world-wise, and street-wise. For three drug-free days and nights he talked to these men—and they reached down into his being and touched him. When I saw him again, he was no longer violent. He said, "Doc, I don't need no more drugs. What I need is a human tranquilizer." He accepted the responsibility for his own life, went on to live at Synanon, a drug rehab program, and led a productive life for at least the next five years, during which we remained in touch.

We must provide that "human tranquilizer" in varying degrees and forms for those who genuinely cannot find one by themselves. And in varying degrees, their life depends on our comfort with their dependency. The small dependent child that is in us all to one extent or another needs to be accepted and assisted at that level, with a mutual clear sight on the goal of making people stand, not alone, but on their own two feet as they make decisions, with us, for the future, near and far.

Alternatives

In seeking alternatives at this stage of our work with the patient, we sometimes require resources or programs outside our immediate competency. Among them may be residential treatment centers and social services such as job training and vocational rehabilitation, Medicaid, foster care, abortion, advice for unwed mothers, welfare, and educational, ecclesiastical, or psychiatric services.

All community resources should be explored, evaluated, utilized, and made known to all members of the therapeutic group. Where the community lacks a given resource, a common, community-wide effort to establish it can weld all of those contributing to it into a strong and purposeful entity (which strengthens the therapeutic community).

Group Support

It is advisable for the acupuncturist to work in an environment with fellow practitioners and those of other healing arts, alternative and otherwise, where clinical experience of others is available for consultation and advice. Group support, in person, by telephone or other rapid methods of correspondence will greatly enhance one's practice and personal comfort in a difficult environment with troubled people with profound disabilities.

Separation and Termination

My concept of the therapeutic relationship is one in which my part is being a "way-station" along the patient's life path, in which I assist patients through an impasse and help them find the right direction to the next "way-station." Although the time at my "station" may last from hours to years, and we may stay in contact for years outside of the "working relationship," it is discontinuous in the sense that passing my way a second or third time may be useful, yet different. Since we are not in this relationship to "win," we can afford not to hold on too tightly; to let people go.

For me the separation is conceived in the context of the finished or unfinished business or the metal phase of "becoming."[18] This involves the transformation of bonds, the ability to move from one bond to another (metal *yang*) and to let go. I would attend to these issues as unfinished business for whichever one of us, the patient or myself or both, for whom the separation is a problem. This attention to the CM aspects would occur in conjunction with a discussion of all aspects of separation and the transformation of bonds.

Discontinuous contact is especially common in work with young people who enter adulthood with a series of projected scenarios and notions about life, each of which needs to be tested despite wise and seasoned reasoning to the contrary. When living out one of these scenarios fails to realize the expected outcome there is a crisis, at which time the person might seek help. If there is a physical component they may end up in an acupuncturist's office where, depending upon the skill of the acupuncturist, the conflict will be uncovered and discussed.

Once that crisis passes the person passes on to testing the next scenario and may withdraw from therapy until that scenario meets the same fate as the first, unless one succeeds. It is extremely important that the patient leaves with the feeling that a contact, a continuation of the relationship, will be welcomed. The best you can do is evoke these dreams and listen to these visions of life, whose pitfalls can be gently suggested. Your sensitive responses will be ignored at first, but not forgotten.

In this regard it is important to realize that any non-harmful relationship with another person has unknown positive consequences. For example, a patient I last saw around 1967–72 wrote the following to my former publisher:

My name is — and I was a patient of Dr. Hammer in 1968 while I attended Southampton College. I know it's been a long time but I would like to thank him for what he has done for me. Can you give me a telephone number or email address so I could contact him? If not please forward this to him. I would like to express my gratitude for what can only be expressed as life-saving.

One can imagine the enormous sense of reassurance to know after so many years that my involvement in this person's life was significant, however brief, in the highly fluid world of drugs and the Vietnamese war. Highly influential in all our lives are surrogate guides and models, beyond our nuclear family, friends, relatives, and teachers, who can change the course of our life. CM practitioners must regard themselves in this very important role as one of those guides.

Either the patient or the practitioner may wish or need to end the therapeutic relationship. It is especially important, when we break the relationship with the patient, to be absolutely clear about our reasons. If they do not involve him or her, he or she must know that we are not leaving because he or she has driven us away. We are also obligated to help establish contact for our patient with a new therapist and to assist in the transition. Usually, parting is best when it is arrived at mutually, with honesty on both sides. This is not always possible.

People are often afraid to offend an authority and therefore leave without notice. It is a good policy to call clients who have missed or cancelled an appointment to encourage them to return one more time, so that they may express directly their reasons for wanting to terminate. Many times this "last" session clears up growing distortions, opens up new vistas in the relationship, and makes for the patient's growth. Sometimes it is the final contact. Always, the client feels better and stronger for having had a direct confrontation with the therapist. As we have already stated, most people are afraid to express disapproval to an authority; having done it once, they are less afraid to do it again.

However parting occurs, it is always possible to leave the door open for future contact, should the need arise.

It is essential in the therapeutic relationship that we observe the basic premise of life, to maintain contact, to get in touch and to keep in touch with the other person. It often requires that we meet some considerable challenges, that we take some risks, that we make sacrifices. But, as long as we maintain contact, we can hope to achieve understanding and change. To the patient, the very effort we expend to maintain contact is a measure of our concern for them. Even the most withdrawn and reluctant person is touched, moved to a new sense of the situation when they see the trouble we are willing to take to reach them and stay with them.

5   Conclusion

I have attempted to outline briefly the principal issues that are involved when two people (or more) come together for the purposes of healing growth and change. Contact has been our basic rule. We know that whatever else may be, people's lives, both in quality and in fact, depend on contact with other people. Our prime consideration is to make and allow for a continuation of contact. No other consideration comes first.

Second, the foundation of that contact is respect. Respect in the therapeutic relationship begins with an acceptance of the patient's maladaptive strategies for staying in contact as the subject of the work, not an expectation that the patient should surrender their lifelong and often unpleasant way of staying "intact" as a condition for being in the therapeutic relationship.

Respect does require that the interaction maintains the patient's best interests in the service of healing, even if an interaction creates friction between the patient and the practitioner ("tough love"). Respect will almost always restore harmony because, as Francis Peabody said, "the secret care of the patient is in caring for the patient," and the patient knows when they are truly cared for.[1]

Third, we have explored the technical aspects that apply, especially, to communication and the principles of listening (input) and feedback or response (output).

Lastly, we have concerned ourselves briefly with the future, near and far, and those issues that relate to mutuality, trial and error, and finally to separation.

The work is difficult, yet basic to healing, indispensable to many, and always worthwhile. It requires commitment, sincerity, humility, respect, and the desire to grow. The outcome, even in what initially appears to be failure, is rewarding to the point of being awesome.

Chinese Medicine (CM) is a medicine that addresses the root cause of problems, not just their physical manifestation; a medicine that treats the whole person, not just the symptoms. The whole person involves the body, mind, and spirit. This is a basic tenet of all traditional medicines. Even modern, materialistically based medicines are increasingly recognizing that one cannot successfully treat one part of a human being in isolation from the rest. The practitioner of either Western or Oriental medicine who consistently ignores and fails to address the emotional and spiritual is a technician and not a true physician.

Terminology of the terms "spirit" and "spiritual" in Chinese Medicine requires clarification. "Spirit" ist evaluated by the sound of the voice, the luster of the skin, the light in the eyes, and posture and movement as well as the response to stress. We are not speaking of "soulful." I give an example of spirit as someone who described herself as lacking in spirit compared with her friend with whom she experienced a serious automobile accident. The friend "became bossy and demanding, while I, on the other hand, went into a deep shell and barely wanted to live."

"Spiritual" on the other hand means a set of individual beliefs and experiences in relation to the cosmos, and while it could occupy a central aspect of therapy, it is generally the province of the religious counselor. "Soulful" means an inward-moving response to life that implies a soft sensitivity to people and the environment. This is a problem only when denial interferes with the ability to experience pain and evaluate danger and is within the province of this book.

This is not a training manual for psychotherapists and counselors. It is intended to convey the fundamental elements of all healing relationships in which all CM practitioners are inevitably involved and to further acquaint practitioners of CM with the nature of what their patients experience when they are referred to a mental health practitioner.

I repeat my earlier assertion that all of the techniques discussed are in the service of advancing "awareness." "Awareness" is a term that summarizes the quest of all esoteric religions as the highest state of consciousness closest to God. It has been my experience that acupuncture is a superb vehicle for enhancing "awareness," and that the acupuncturist is in a unique place in the pantheon of healers to combine this art with those techniques described in this book to advance this cause.

Section II

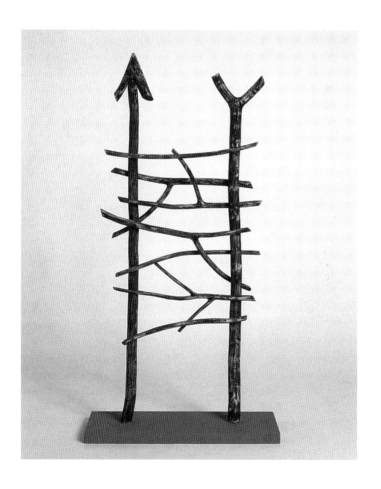

Section II—Questions and Answers

The ultimate value of this book is the degree to which it helps the practitioner to deal with their day-to-day challenges in the clinic. I have therefore asked practitioners who I have been able to reach over the years about their clinical dilemmas and have received a number of replies that have been consolidated into some fundamental questions listed over the following pages, together with my responses. Some of those who responded also provided answers that are quoted when appropriate. I want to express my appreciation to all of them.

Chinese Medicine (CM) has the tools to diagnose and therefore manage the individual who has a disease. The answers given below are general and generic and must be considered in the context of the individual with whom the events are unfolding and for which an answer is sought. Some of the answers are embodied with the basic principles of the therapeutic relationship covered in Section I of this book.

Perhaps the universal answer to all our questions is answered in the age-old admonition, "physician know thyself." This may not be very easy and no one *has* to work this way, even if I believe it is the most rewarding way.

Betrayal and Attachment: What Can Practitioners Do When a Patient Resists Treatment that is Working?

Observation from Correspondent

"K," a chronically ill patient, to whom I had given all of my attention and skill and beyond for several years, wrote unexpectedly telling me that she had found a better acupuncturist from whom she is receiving more help than I had ever given her. Under my care she had reportedly improved significantly and yet this sudden disaffection accompanied by a diminishment of my ability and service has been very painful and made me very angry. I see her as a borderline personality and have the feeling that I will hear from her again.

Answer by Dr. Hammer

As I read the saga about your patient "K" I experienced the anguish of the betrayal. It is impossible not to want to give back the hurt one receives when one opens one's heart and a knife is the reply. The dilemma is that one cannot do this work well without an open heart, love, and respect, and therefore one is always vulnerable. It is important to assess each person in order to know what to expect and be prepared, and yet, as we see, this is an imperfect process.

What is meant by an "open heart"? For me it means being completely with and almost "as" that person while I am with them. Athletes call this "being in the zone." Out of the "zone" I am another person that I know as "me." But still, who is so perfectly confident, especially with work that does not have a linear measurable outcome, that the rejection by another is not in varying degrees profoundly painful? It may be some comfort to realize that even if "K" is receiving more help with this new therapist now, that person is building on the hard work that you have done previously.

I resist the temptation to ascribe mental and personality conditions to patients, especially after a painful separation, because in our society a diagnosis of mental illness can become a compensatory comforting derogation. However, with regard to being prepared as mentioned above, it can be useful to make a cautious assessment of what to expect. There are no two people with any diagnosis, mental or physical, who are exactly the same. With the tools of CM we can delineate an individual apart from their disease entity and treat the person as well as the illness.

A person with a "borderline personality" may be either so defeated that they must bring to others the same humiliation they feel, or be so angry at authority that they must defeat it. These people will undermine the practitioner in endless ways, through non-compliance, through self-destructive behavior and, if all else fails, by suddenly abandoning the therapy, even if it costs them the benefit they already feel. These individuals usually do this without notice, transmitting directly or indirectly to the practitioners that they are poor at their job and the preference for another practitioner. This happens especially if the patient senses the caring investment made by the practitioner and thus the potential to hurt.

For health care providers of all kinds, borderline personalities are the most difficult to treat because they cannot sufficiently trust a relationship with an authority figure to form a working bond. The relationship must be accepted at best as discontinuous. If the practitioner can contain their hurt and disappointment, the borderline patient might be back, and will leave again without warning in the same manner. Over long periods of time, these patterns, if they can be endured, sometimes succumb to the endless tests for love. One's boundaries must be maintained with impassionate, clearly communicated assessments of the uncertainty of the relationship, acknowledging the patient's ability to hurt, together with firm expectations for what would be a more successful strategy for a meaningful outcome.

Obviously the patient felt drawn to open herself to you more strongly than she could bear. The human mind always makes "rational" explanations to itself for its irrational impulses, and her modus operandi for this purpose is clearly deprecation. I wonder about her long-term relationship with another woman considering the "intensity shifting from side to side," but I assume you have sufficient evidence to support this. If she is homosexual she may have another reason to attempt to undermine your confidence, which she would not with a new therapist who is also homosexual.

In retrospect, there were reasons to question the veracity of her dissatisfaction. The suppressed quality on her pulse points to her being on substances (medications) at this time that she denies. Your diagnosis of borderline personality is supported by the shape of her tongue (hammer shape), a sign of very early personality damage, which is always associated with this kind of diagnosis. Though we cannot be certain, rough vibration on the entire pulse is sometimes a sign of guilt for something she may have a profound fear of being discovered, or a severe emotional shock.

The saying that "misery loves company" is especially true for those who are failing in life and seeing others failing likewise is a sense of comfort and a source of power for the otherwise inwardly powerless. The patient has, by deprecating the practitioner and the therapy, the potential power to diminish another. Therapy is a relatively safe place to do this. Furthermore, a successful collaboration between practitioner and patient invites an intimacy that may threaten the patient, who must create a distance in one of many ways. Denial of success and otherwise derogating the practitioner and the work obviates the threat of closeness.

In the end we must face the fact that we are hurt, and plumb the depths of our vulnerability as a challenge to our own growth.

How Should Practitioners Talk to Patients about Psychological Problems and Processes in the Context of CM Thinking and Treatment?

Answer by Dr. Hammer

Example

Condition

A 73-year-old male patient (Mr. Q) came with symptoms of palpitations in the middle of the night and an increasing ache from certain activities, especially walking his dog and bicycling to the market. Furthermore, it occurred on his way to the market and not on the way home. He experienced no pain going up and down the stairs in his home and while playing actively with his grandchild. The ache was primarily in his left chest, shoulder, and arm, but sometimes migrated to his right shoulder and right hip, though less often. It was his conviction that he had severe heart disease.

His pulse rate was slow (52 beats/minute) and an examination of the vessels revealed ropy (twisting and standing out from the arm) and leather (hard) qualities. These are signs that the vessels are hardening, deficient of *yin* and that there is an obstruction to circulation that in turn would make the heart have to work harder. There was a full-overflowing wave, a sign of heat in the blood ordinarily associated with hypertension, but with no elevation in blood pressure. This is a condition associated with very long-term exercise, perhaps by participating in vigorous sport, beyond a person's basic energy, as explained in *Chinese Pulse Diagnosis: A Contemporary Approach*[1] and by Dr. Shen.[2] (This "*qi* wild" condition is discussed in the section on the hollow and hollow full-overflowing qualities in Chapter 8 of *Chinese Pulse Diagnosis*.) The drying out of the intima and media of the vessels in this case is due to lack of nourishment, rather than heat.

Exercising beyond one's energy over a long period of time causes the *yin* (nourishing blood and *qi*) flowing in the center of the vessel to be depleted and separated from the activating *yang qi* at the surface of the vessel, thereby depriving the vessel walls of the nourishment needed to maintain their flexibility. **Over-exercise causes gradual shrinking of *yin* blood—using up more than can be replaced—while the heart pumps harder to maintain circulation, causing the walls to remain distended.**

I have observed this combination several times in recent years, and once found it in a 60-year-old marathon runner subsequently diagnosed with Parkinson disease. I would speculate that this may involve impaired circulation to the brain related to the alterations in the blood vessels indicated by the ropy and yielding quality. However, I do not have enough clinical experience with this quality to cogently address the issue of associated syndromes.

Mr. Q was also marathon runner practicing up to 6 miles a day for most of his adult life in addition to other exercise. The leather quality on Mr. Q's pulse and a simultaneous thick blood condition suggests that two processes were at work. One is described above involving the depletion of blood and separation of vessel from circulating blood, and the other is an excess heat in the blood for reasons to be explained.

For many years, Mr. Q has had many escalating frustrations and rage in his life that he cannot express and represses. Increasingly he feels impotent to control his own life, in which all of his lifelong plans for retirement are totally frustrated. The excess heat in his liver in order to move the stagnant *qi* associated with repression has entered the blood as a way of protecting the liver. However, in addition to the vessel walls being depleted of blood, they have also experienced a high degree of heat that has hardened (vulcanized) the intimae and media of the vessels.

Feedback to Patient

The object here is to relate the patient's condition to his life experience and lifestyle. It must be clearly stated that to do so requires repeated explanations for those not familiar with the medicine until the connections are clear.

Given the symptoms of palpitations and chest ache in areas associated by the layperson with a heart affliction, it was not a great leap from this awareness to a connection with the issue of his circulation and the condition of his vessels.

The idea that a machine that overworks, overheats, and how that heat vulcanized his vessel walls and depleted them of fluid was another easy step. That Mr. Q was this machine that was overworking through years of marathon running was also not a difficult step, despite being told for years by allopathic physicians that marathons would prevent the coronary occlusion he had just experienced.

We then came to the issue of his frustration, about which he became more voluble. Framed conceptually as a build up of heat trying to overcome his acknowledged repression, and periodically blowing off steam as with the steam in a boiler when the pressure gets to be too high, was easy to envisage. Envisaging that the escaping steam (heat) contained in his body would travel to vulnerable areas was, further, an easy step. Even easier to see from what we had already discussed was that his heart was vulnerable.

It was not a big step from here for him to see that when he experienced joy, as with his grandson, or was on his way home from the market to the "safety" of his home that he loved, that no amount of activity resulted in his ache. This brought home the association of his "heart aches" with his emotional life, especially as he was also acutely aware of his lifelong social anxiety and his relative social comfort when alone or with his family.

The "attacking" excess heat from the liver creates stagnation and chaos in the heart, interfering with the heart's ability to circulate blood efficiently both peripherally and to the coronary arteries. From common knowledge, he had already correctly associated the chest and left arm aches with decreased coronary blood flow. The connection with his repressed emotions, the effect on his liver, and the consequences to his heart now made increasing sense to him.

This would also explain the palpitations at night. This is the time when the liver is at the height of its activity and therefore, the escaping heat has its greatest stimulating effect on his heart. It is also the time when the blood is stored in the liver and concomitantly less available to the heart. The heart must then work harder to dissipate the aimless dysfunction of heat from the liver. Since there is no exertion while asleep, the consequences are palpitations (an overworking heart) rather than an ache.

How Can Practitioners Guide and/or Support Patients through Psychological Events and Challenges?

This includes emotional and cognitive responses to treatment that are sometimes dramatic, intense, and distressing to patient and practitioner; for example, a crisis related to past abuse and the question of whether so a so-called healing crisis is useful or a risk to the patient.

Answer from Correspondents

The following statement, provided by a correspondent, exquisitely expresses my own sentiment:

> *[By] relying on that in myself that is faithful, trustworthy, and open, and trying to communicate that naturally. Patients understand that even if it's just the "Ten Questions."*

Another correspondent contributed the following:

> *Through my own living I have had experiences that help me to listen, suspend judgment, relate to, and offer options that have worked for me in my own experiences.*

Answer by Dr. Hammer

Both correspondents' answers would be among my own.

The ability to accompany and stay with a patient into what I called in *Dragon Rises—Red Bird Flies*,[3] the "descent into hell," depends on the capacity to benefit from one's own descent, and on the nature of that descent, the patient's and one's own.

The principles outlined in Section I of this book, especially authenticity (see Chapter 1), are essential. The patient should know your limitations with regard to the immediate issue, and your absolute commitment to finding them help in a safe environment for those things that you cannot provide. Any deviation from that authenticity will destroy the relationship that can otherwise survive the acknowledged boundaries of one's competence.

This competence does not depend on training. When I practiced as a psychiatrist-psychoanalyst, I received frequent calls from highly trained colleagues who referred patients "who had no self," jargon for my colleagues' inability to deal with their terror of psychosis, which for some reason I did not share.

Any "healing crisis" that lasts more than a few days is something more serious and should be addressed clinically rather than advising the patient to endure in the interests of therapy.

How Can Practitioners Recognize and Deal with a Situation that is Beyond Their Knowledge or Capacity to Handle and Requires Assistance and Referral to Other Health Care Providers Including Hospitalization?

Answer from Correspondent

We have to define our own comfort level and boundaries as far as counseling is concerned. If a person is asking for help with their mental or emotional state I talk to them about the relationship of energy imbalance on the physical and spirit level but state plainly to them that I am not a counselor and they need to consider getting help from a psych professional along with the energetic work that we may do together. This, of course, depends on the degree of distress they are in. Most frequently in my experience if a patient is having great difficulty coping they already have a counselor or psychiatrist.

There have been a couple of instances where I have called a patient's counselor because they were in a crisis and needed immediate help. We need to know when a person is beyond our capability.

It so happens that the office I work in shares space with a counseling group so I have always been able to get advice or help easily. I think all acupuncturists should develop a contact line to someone or a group who can help in this way.

Answer by Dr. Hammer

Again, authenticity is the key ingredient. If you experiences anxiety or panic when faced with the patient's issues, you must acknowledge that to yourself and communicate to the patient your mutual need to find another resource to cope with the situation.

You will avoid the risk of alienating the patient if you take full responsibility for not being able to cope with the situation, while also being committed to finding a safe solution as quickly as the situation requires. If this requires heroic measures such as hospitalization this is usually accomplished by simply stating the obvious that: "You are telling me, not I you, that you are in deep trouble, and I am telling you that as much as I want to, I am not qualified to provide the help you need. Do you have any other suggestions?"

If the person denies the need for hospitalization that you and others clearly see, I have found it useful to look at the patient very directly and calmly say, "Let us forget what the others say about your condition. You and I both know that that is where you need to be for now." I personally have never had anyone resist this recommendation, and I have had hundreds of experiences in the Admitting Office of Bellevue Psychiatric Hospital in New York City and in my practice over the past 35 years.

If all else fails, have the patient hospitalized either from your office, if it feels safe, or after they leave if the patient is potentially violent. As for the threat of violence, it is best to stay calm and concede the danger you feel to the patient as I explain in the answer to the next question on page 98. An outward show of fear is only going to increase the patient's fear and the likelihood of striking out. Someone has to stay in control if there is a possibility that the patient cannot.

How Can Practitioners Deal Constructively with a Patient's Distrust, Skepticism, Disappointment, Criticism, and Anger Directed at Them?

Answer by Dr. Hammer

I find myself returning repeatedly to the issue of authenticity. I will give you an example.

Example

An African-American man was referred to me by a psychiatrist. The patient was a huge man. At the end of the first session, as he was leaving he placed his hands on either side of the door to my office, announcing that he was going to destroy it, because he had been denigrated—the referring psychiatrist who was treating his wife lived in a more upscale part of town (Fifth Avenue) and he was sent to see a psychiatrist living in a less upscale part of town (Central Park West).

I stared at him for a moment and then spontaneously acknowledged that if this was his intention that I had every reason to believe from his size and anger that he could do it, easily. I made no move to oppose him or call for help. We stared at each other for a few moments and suddenly he relaxed, turned around and left. I realistically acknowledged his power and this enhanced his self-esteem sufficiently that he did not to have to act to prove it. I continued to see this man for many years and continued a correspondence for years after his life and mine took separate geographical paths.

Within the context of the therapy, the patient's negative feelings can cause hurt and fear and this must be acknowledged so that they know that they have power. At the same time they must also see that though they can hurt, their negative feeling (as differentiated from action) cannot destroy. The practitioner must acknowledge the hurt that they do not like, while pointing out that they are still there functioning. The practitioner can feel the patient's power while becoming less afraid of it.

How Should Practitioners Handle the Cessation of Treatment and/or Relationship?

See the final section in Chapter 4 on "Separation and Termination."

How Should Practitioners Cope with "Difficult" Patients?

For example, this could include a patient who is always trying to control or dominate the practitioner and the process regardless of the stated or agreed objective of treatment.

Answer by Dr. Hammer

The following, taken from Chapter 6 of my book, *Dragon Rises—Red Bird Flies*,[3] seems relevant here:

> *Except in instances of "possession" (control by external forces), human beings strive to contact others within a context of positive emotion.*

> *Human experience may not always allow the positive emotions to flourish; in many circumstances, negative or hostile contact may be all that is possible and, paradoxically, may be life-sustaining. If life requires this as an enduring condition, negativity becomes a way of life.*

> *Negativity is maladaptive and it ultimately fails. Negativity is annoying, and our understandable response is to destroy or contain it. This is a natural reaction but is rarely therapeutic, except under very special circumstances (in a context of proven love). The therapeutic community, since the dawn of our era, has experienced this negativity as "resistance" and has reacted to it with professionally rationalized and distilled hostility, known in the literature as "analyzing the resistance," "shock treatment," or "chemical restraints."*

As health practitioners we are of value to the people who consult us only if we can offer them something significantly different from the usual response. Of course, we recognize and acknowledge the negative in all its destructiveness. However …

We are needed for our ability to recognize the positive quest for contact beneath the negative emotions and behavior; this need is especially great for those who have already come to disdain themselves.

This is the beginning of a 'new experience' with someone who is reliably more concerned with finding, and responding to, the positive rather than the negative in them; with someone nourishing rather than condemning; with someone capable of putting, at least temporarily, another person's needs ahead of his or her own.

Only as we allow a 'new experience' and provide a new model can our contact with our patients be a truly healing, growing, therapeutic experience.

In the service of staying "intact" by maintaining ineluctable "contact," people interact often maladaptively according to how they learned to stay intact in their formative years with their dysfunctional family of origin or with a dysfunctional surrogate. This is what they learned and it is only through the ability to separate the innate talent for positive contact from the negative (which ultimately alienates people), that people can gradually become adaptive, nourishing people, rather than draining and disruptive of even one's own best interests.

There is a principle in re-evaluation therapy that says that "people do things *that* annoy us, not *to* annoy us." While demonstrating our patience and concern, we can simultaneously confront people with behavior that is not in anyone's best interest and point out the destructive consequences to them of their negativity.

How Should Practitioners Handle Issues of Money and Missing Appointments?

I offer the patient one missed appointment without payment during our tenure if it is to be long term, that is, more than 10 sessions. If the fee is beyond their ability to pay I will reduce it if possible, and sometimes I will see those impecunious patients during my lunch hour for a lower fee or free of charge.

We must remember that people cannot change just by making an appointment to see us, and that they must necessarily bring their emotional baggage with them. So, if they are consistently late in order to test our commitment to them and/or recieve the usual angry reaction that to them is "contact," we can acknowledge that one of our objectives is to make this alienating behavior unnecessary. In the meantime, if they are late, they simply have less time in which to benefit from the therapy.

How Can Practitioners Handle Inappropriate Sexual Approaches by Patients?

Answer by Dr. Hammer

I covered this subject briefly in the section on Touching (Therapeutic) in Chapter 4.

It is important to acknowledge one's attraction to the patient if such exists and that for both there is a sacrifice to be made in the interests of their mutually stated goals of therapy. If those goals have changed for the patient, they would have to accept that they have not changed for the therapist; the therapist's commitment is to do no harm, which such a relationship could entail, even if the therapy is suspended.

If both parties are serious, there should be a suspension of contact for at least 6 months as a test of the nature of the relationship and its durability.

How Should Practitioners Handle Friendship with Patients In and Out of the Clinical Setting?

Answer by Dr. Hammer

Friendships are very delicate relationships, especially between men. It is a difficult situation when you fail to help someone you care about, and then wonder if the relationship can be repaired afterward.

I have observed that students in the clinic at Dragon Rises College of Oriental Medicine in Florida who treat friends find them much more difficult to work with than other patients.

I rarely succeeded in treating friends even while following all of the principles mentioned here and in Section I of this book. Avoiding all such commitments is difficult, however, and I now begin treatment by placing all of the dangers "on the table" as soon as is practical.

How Should Practitioners Handle Patients Who Put Them on a Pedestal?

Answer by Dr. Hammer

Since we all have feet of clay, the only place one can go from a pedestal is down. One should be gracious in accepting praise, while being clear that the praise is meaningful to you only when you have demonstrated real achievement. This should be followed by an explanation of the danger to the work when you inevitably fall from the pedestal and an inquiry about the source of the adulation, which is doomed to fail and lead to disillusionment.

For one's own information, being familiar with borderline and "oral" personalities [1] is possibly helpful in understanding the expectation for a perfect all-delivering "parent" and the rage when that fails to materialize.

How Should Practitioners Deal with People Who Are Insufficient in Specific Life Functions, Which in Themselves Will Create Further Emotional Problems?

Answer by Dr. Hammer

Introduction

In the long run, we hope, as mentioned in the section on "Dependence, Independence, and Initiative" in Chapter 4, that each of us will stand on his or her own two feet. But, at the different stages of a therapeutic relationship, some degree of leaning and dependency is necessary, especially during transitions. The trick is to let people lean so that they can grow stronger (not weaker). Still, they must lean and we must deal with our problem, if we have one, with dependency.

Dependency has poor press in our "pull yourself up by the bootstraps" culture. We are in constant fear of nurture as undermining self-reliance in our children and our patients and speak more easily of "tough love" than love. Nevertheless, this repugnance in our society reflected in the psychotherapeutic world is entirely illogical.

Acting for the patient, when it is clear to me that they truly cannot act for themselves, has often had dramatic effects in terms of teaching by example, on the rare occasions people use my intervention to escape facing the issue. I am not fearful of a dependency that I see as a necessity in the course of individuation, a dependency that failed to lead to growth and maturity during the appropriate stage of development and must be revisited within a therapeutic relationship.

One of the ways that practitioners feel uncomfortable with the dependency of their patients is the latter's inability to take the initiative for themselves. Sometimes this involves the simplest things, such as the patient calling the telephone company when they move house. Sometimes it involves more complicated procedures such as applications for a job. I have assumed these ego functions frequently, in the service of our having the time to build the terrain, the missing pieces, that render the patient ultimately able to function on their own.

Many of the people CM practitioners see are those whose adaptations for survival are less acceptable either to society or even to themselves. The young man we will discuss below escaped into drugs in order to live with that part of himself that would have been intolerable to his ego, his fear of fighting for what he believed. He would have had to look in the mirror of his own mind and of the society he lives in and see the word "coward," and being unable to tolerate that, escaped condemnation either through mind-numbing substances, a living death, or ultimate death. For years he dressed and behaved the image of "tough," to reassure himself and discourage attack from an ever-threatening world. Such people are the truly and rationally dependent ones. They are the ones who need to lean on us until our therapy gives them the strength to lean upon themselves.

The following is an elaboration of the example in the section on "Dependence, Independence, and Initiative" in Chapter 4 of the proactive role that I have played with people whose egos ("terrain") are not yet stable or sufficient to perform certain functions that interfere with their goals in life and our efforts to achieve them.

Example

The young man in question, a 39-year-old carpenter, had been abusing substances since he was 14 years old, beginning with alcohol and excessive use of marihuana, cocaine "if nothing else is available," and intravenous heroin for the past 9 years. Recently he felt the need for more, especially heroin, "to feel good."

He was beginning to realize that he was almost 40 years old and was unproductive, unmotivated, without direction or aspiration, inadequate at work and in relationships, isolated, and remorseful of a wasted life with no energy. He stated that "I am a creative person with no outlet, guilty due to not working, sleeping all day to avoid awareness and staying awake all night when I am not expected to do anything (work) except watch TV."

The patient has grandiose ideas of what he sees himself doing for a just society, recognizing that he is not accomplishing much in real life. He is a hero in many fantasies. He confides that he inflates himself in how he walks and talks to give the appearance of strength, while inwardly feeling weak and not able to stand up for his ideals. He is at the same time the interminably and fanatically arch critique of a society in which he feels a victim.

He describes high ideals for society, especially for peace, and yet he does not wish to be involved in life unless he can do so without straining himself. In this context, saving the environment was one of his principle preoccupations. He disdains ordinary approaches to solving his problems such as AA, and even my work, as all on a low spiritual level. He seeks a higher spiritual guidance, apparently in the "New Age" fashion it seems, rather than through the pain and hard work involved in the daily struggle of life. His goal is to feel strong enough to work and live out his ideals.

He was described by his mother, who was traumatized early and throughout the pregnancy, as vulnerable from birth and unable to talk until he was 3 years old, requiring protection throughout his childhood. Diagnostically there was severe liver *qi* deficiency and retained pathogen, severe kidney *qi* deficiency and separation of *yin* and *yang* of the heart. It was clear from the beginning that so many years of the cold substances, marihuana and heroin, that his ability to put his thoughts into action were severely impaired. Where would we begin?

Based on past experience in similar circumstances, I realized that he did not have the ability to move out alone from his current morass and enjoy whatever help was available until he could break the vicious cycle described above. Work was available to him as a carpenter if he could get to it. I proposed that since he "did not have a liver" to provide planning, decisions, and a direction in order to break the impasse of night-day reversal that I would "loan" him my liver. We agreed that I would call him every morning at 7:00 a.m, plan the work for the day, and at first check with him in the evening. This began and lasted for several months, taking a total of about 2 minutes of my time per day. He began to work productively, reversed his night–day schedule, and gradually reduced his use of drugs.

He left working with me after a few more months because I was not spiritually advanced enough for him, and took excursions literally into the wilderness. Nevertheless, with no other therapy I am aware of, he has rarely taken drugs and has continued to work. Nothing has changed about his view of the world or of his ability to intervene on its behalf, while still loudly proclaiming its leaders to be scoundrels. We see each other occasionally on the street and hug.

Sharing and Decision-making

Of particular importance with regard to the "how" of the "therapeutic relationship" is the sharing of responsibility for decisions, including separation discussed in Chapters 3 and 4. In the model we are attempting to live out with another person, we collaborate and still retain our individuality. Our exploration, however heated and intimate, however complex it may become, is mutual. (Dictionaries define mutuality as "done, felt, or with regard to the other," "with the same feelings," or "with the same relationship to each other.")

Our object is to help our patient find *their* way. If we lose sight of this, we defeat one significant purpose of our exploration—to pay respect to the person who has lost his or her self-respect. We will have forgotten that our respect for their unique being is their bridge to restored self-respect. The challenge here is to retain the mutual aspects of our relations while helping them formulate decisions specifically fitted to their needs.

When we have achieved enough insight to delineate the problem before us by mutual agreement, and understand it reasonably well in terms of the patient's innate needs and conflicts, we are ready to make decisions. In the beginning stages of the "therapeutic relationship," it is helpful to explore with the patient the direction of their life and the possible, or probable, consequences of its present course. As they verbalize their present direction and its consequences, they can help clarify their motivation.

Somewhere along the way, the patient, with the acupuncturist's help, must make decisions about real-life problems. They are developing realistic goals, goals consistent with their needs, and, although the acupuncturist has played a critical role in this process of growth, he or she has not imposed these goals. They are the patient's own, evolved through changes in them.

In orienting him- or herself, the patient asks him- or herself some questions: should I remain at home or begin my move out on my own? Do I need a period away from school to find myself, in myself and in the world, before I give learning a serious place in my life? Should I continue to associate with people who need me to share their destructive way of life—as, for example, with drugs? Would they want me or help me if I wanted something different from what they want? Are they really my friends? What is a friend?

These decisions are occasions for initiating new and more productive patterns of living. Almost always they are fraught with deep anxiety. This is because they are ventures into the unknown. We all fear the unknown: trying new patterns of behavior, expressing previously buried feelings—these are frightening unless we have a great deal of experience in exploring unknowns; few of us are so adventurous. There are occasions for all of us when we do not wish to be alone and wish to share with another, sometimes necessarily the practitioner.

How Can Practitioners Provide Nourishment to People Who Lacked it Early in Life?

Question from Correspondent

How can I, a (fairly) young, mostly hairy male practitioner offer the kind of nourishment to those patients who lacked nourishment early in life, and who seem to be perpetually looking for someone to take care of them?

Answer by Dr. Hammer

Listening, using all of the principles described in this book, is the ground on which this nourishment can grow, especially the willingness to support the patient as described before (see questions on pp. 95 and 103 above and Chapter 4, p. 37) concerning issues of dependency.

The investment of the practitioner is a function of the love of the medicine and the love of the patient for whom one has an inner need to help. Without words, the practitioner's love is transmitted energetically to the patient through presence, and through the choice of points one uses to treat the patient, for example, using moxa on ren-8 is a recognition of the need for the vital maternal nourishment, as is using the formula, *Shi Quan Da Bu Wan* (Pill of Ten Powerful Tonics).

Seeing the person and reflecting what one sees, hearing the person and responding to what one hears, recognizing the best and accepting and helping with the worst is all the nourishment needed. And this can be given even by people with "hairy legs."

How Should Practitioners Respond to Issues of Transference and Counter-transference [2]

This also includes affection for and dislike of patients, and how to utilize either negative or positive emotional forces that grow and emerge in people in the service of healing and/or problem-solving.

Answer by Dr. Hammer

Most of what we have already discussed can be considered counter-transference issues except with regard to sexual attraction by the therapist for the patient. What we have not addressed is the situation where the practitioner genuinely dislikes or is made anxious by the patient.

These are reactions that can be separate or directly connected in as much as we dislike what makes us uncomfortable. To repeat our dictum, the first order is "physician know thyself." We can explore or ask others to help us explore the nature of this disaffection, with us as the subject. This can be part of our growth as people and professionals.

Self-exploration may take more time than is practical in a clinical situation where the dislike and discomfort is clearly interfering with the work, at which time you can be frank with the patient, explaining that you do not feel competent to address their problem and could refer them to another practitioner. Do this when you have an alternative to offer, and take full responsibility, explaining that it is regretfully your limitation and not theirs. Let them express their reaction and support them through their pain until a transition is achieved, validating that this could feel like a rejection and a diminishment and absorbing any anger that you acknowledge is understandable.

From the clinician's perspective it may be wise to terminate the work, but not the commitment to explore one's reaction.

How Can Practitioners Extract the Essential or Correct from the Less Important or Incorrect?

Observation from Correspondent

I noticed during the Pulse Intensive Workshop that even when someone said something obviously or egregiously incorrect, you managed to correct him/ her without necessarily contradicting him/her from the start. It is as if you were able to discern the element of truth in the comment, and emphasize that in relation to the rest of the statement. Then the element of truth was highlighted and, lo and behold, you had said something very instructive. Now this is a teaching scenario and not a therapeutic one, but I think it could be extrapolated into a therapeutic context. It involves discerning the essential from the less important, asking the right questions, and developing skill in communicating with another person in a non-judgmental and affirming fashion. All of which seems vital to "asking."

Answer by Dr. Hammer

Every person brings their innate God-given and acquired talent to their life situation. That talent is always there and the task is to separate the gold from the dross, the talent from its misuse, almost always unintentional. There is evil in the world. Our job is to recognize and acknowledge it, to isolate it from doing harm, and then see what else is there. As one approach, I identify where people's disturbing perceptions are correct and incorrect as the example below illustrates.

Example

A patient expresses one day that he thinks you do not like him. One can examine this in two ways, as an issue of perception and an issue of interpretation.

Perception

Upon questioning, he says he can identify an angry look on your face. Ask him what in your face indicates that you are angry. It could be that you did not shave, or certain lines in your face are exaggerated by lack of sleep, or if you are female, a change in make-up. Examine your face and confirm or validate what he correctly perceived or if you cannot confirm it on your own inspection, ask him to point to the offending signs, which then can be examined together. If you still cannot see them, just suggest that you are seeing different things that are equally valid if not consensual.

Interpretation

If you were indeed angry that day for some reason you can point out that their perception was correct, that you have been angry, explaining the reason as far as you feel comfortable (for example, problem with the computer, your spouse, and so on) and point out that they can trust their perceptive skill but must question their interpretation, which they center on themselves. Repetition of this process gradually leads the patient to trust their perceptions and question their interpretations.

How Can Practitioners Extract the Positive from What Seems Negative—Native Brilliance or a Skill Acquired?

Observation from Correspondent

I understand that experience plays a huge part in the development of this skill. I feel that some guidelines would ease the transition from neophyte to seasoned "interrogator." Another issue, of course, which highlights the difference in your experience and that of the average acupuncturist, is precisely the question of scope. As interested as I am (which is extremely interested) in helping patients through emotional/psychological/spiritual difficulties, I don't ever want to overstep my bounds.

Answer by Dr. Hammer

One acquires this skill with conjoint practice under the supervision of one already adroit and experienced. Apprenticeship and repetition is the answer for those whose life experience and inclination brings them to share other people's inner life. "Knowing thyself" is indispensable to the skill.

I return to my frequently repeated assertion that respect, authenticity, caring, and the development of the ability to be both with, and "be," the patient, are the essential ingredients. These are elaborated on in Section I of this book.

Listening is an art that depends on hearing with the "third ear," as well as looking with the "third eye" (see Chapter 4), especially to find what the patient is avoiding saying or showing. There are many approaches to this, including questions one can ask, such as: "If there was one thing that you could change about yourself and about your life …" or, "How are you a problem to yourself?"

People from infancy to death need to be seen, to be heard, and to have a constructive response. And they want to be seen and heard by someone whose passion it is to heal. Again, look for and identify the positive and separate it from the negative.

Should Practitioners Use Western Counseling Techniques and Approaches, or CM, or Both?

Answer by Dr. Hammer

While the results of CM diagnostic techniques can be translated into insights useful to the emotional life of a person, the techniques of Western counseling are elucidated in this text and are no different for a patient in CM than in any other therapeutic situation. People are, after all, people. However, there are some qualifying considerations. One is culture. If one is treating people from outside one's own culture one must recognize that issues that are relatively easy for one culture to address, might be intolerable to people from another culture.

Examples

For example, I did a bioenergetic workshop in London in 1971 in which one partici-pant, a large man, who acknowledged his anger, could not express it by pounding a pillow and instead recited the following poem:

Out of the night that covers me,
Black as the Pit from pole to pole,
I thank whatever gods may be
For my unconquerable soul.

In the fell clutch of circumstance
I have not winced nor cried aloud.
Under the bludgeonings of chance
My head is bloody, but unbowed.

Beyond this place of wrath and tears
Looms but the Horror of the shade,
And yet the menace of the years
Finds, and shall find, me unafraid.

It matters not how strait the gate,
How charged with punishments the scroll,
I am the master of my fate:
I am the captain of my soul.

("Invictus," 1875, by William Earnest Henley[5])

In China in 1981, shortly after the "official" end of the Cultural Revolution, I encountered tremendous repressed rage in the patients in the hospital where I worked. This would have been a quick death sentence for anyone who dared to express it, even to members of family or close friends, because everyone was spying on each other. Another example might include the danger of encouraging a Moslem woman to express openly or act upon her sexual or even educational longing. The list of such cautions is as endless as the difference in cultures.

How Can Practitioners Safely Combine Lifestyle Management and CM Diagnosis?

Answer by Dr. Hammer

On p. 106, we looked at some examples of the difficult issues that people from different cultures or religions may have to deal with. In matters of lifestyle management techniques there are also cautions for the practitioner, as the following example shows.

Example

An elderly woman from a lower to middle class, devoutly Catholic background and little education, with 15 pregnancies and surgical intervention on almost every organ in her body came to an acupuncturist for the treatment of back pain. She was advised at the first session to begin practicing an esoteric form of meditation. This woman lost her formerly tightly held boundaries within the parameters of her religion and gradually became psychotic.

I have seen this happen frequently among young people in the 1960s and 1970s, drawn into esoteric practices by knee-jerk "New Age" counselors to address their emotional problems. These people, already with chaotic psyches, frequently emerged psychotic from these unguided immersions into their consciousness, when they were meant, diagnostically, to be led into a reality-testing, ego-enhancing, grounding therapy.

CM diagnosis, especially a sophisticated pulse system,[4] is meant to be a guide to the stability of a person's mental–emotional–spiritual condition. Without going into detail here, signs of a *qi* wild condition, multiple separations of *yin* and *yang*, chaotic rhythms, spinning beans and split pulses [3], to mention a few, can conduct the practitioner to the need for an ego-based approach rather than towards explorations of hidden conflicts.

Here I subscribe to a correspondent's thoughts when he said:

> *I have found that strength of body and mind makes a person more tolerant to emotional difficulty, and emotional difficulty can offer our most vital opportunity for growth. I have been very influenced by your teachings on the importance of cultivating emotional and physical strength, and I have found this to be extremely important in observing myself and others. Whenever I treat someone with needles and herbs I look for ways to strengthen them when possible.*

The correspondent is pointing the way to preparing the way for a person to develop a foundation, a center, and a way of reaching out that would enable them to benefit from meditative work rather than be further disorganized. We make the correct diagnosis first, we employ the appropriate corrective strengthening therapy second, and then with the patient we assess their readiness for a particular road to follow. It was common in my practice for people to tell *me* when they felt ready to move on into spiritual practices with practitioners other than me.

When Should Practitioners Inform Important Others, Spouse, Parents, Relatives, and Other Therapists?

Answer by Dr. Hammer

As part of the original contract I tell people from the very beginning that what occurs within my office is confidential, to never be revealed to any other person except upon the patient's request and consent. I add that the one exception is if in my opinion it is necessary to share decisions involving life and death such as the threat of violence to others or themselves.

How Should Practitioners Advise Patients Who Are Doing Too Many Things, Seeing Too Many Practitioners?

Answer by Dr. Hammer

I suggest to patients that they come to me after they have tried everything else and that once we work together they will forgo any other treatment until we agree to stop. I explain that most illness is the result of physiological chaos and that minimizing that chaos in their lives, in our work, and in their bodies and minds is an ineluctable condition for healing. (And there is always the old saying that "too many cooks spoil the broth.")

This dictum applies to anything that involves our mutual work. While I might not terminate the therapy, keeping in mind that people cannot change a lifetime of negative behavior, I will make it clear how they are undermining their own treatment goals. With the clear admonition, as my teacher Dr. Shen would say, sitting back in his chair with his finger pointing at the patient and in a very clear loud voice, "Your fault, not mine." (Several examples of such situations were submitted by a correspondent, such as "depressed patients who are on medications and try to stop the drugs before they get benefit from acupuncture then crash, and patients who want to get pregnant and won't wait until they regain fertility then get frustrated.")

How Can Practitioners Recognize Who is at Risk?

The following are some warning signs of impending danger:
- sudden changes in behavior and mood:
  - as observed in the clinic and towards the practitioner;
  - as reported with significant others including employers;
- obsessed preoccupation with a subject (possessed):
  - dreams of death;
  - preoccupation with death.

For example, one young man's wife left him to live with his best friend, at which time he was obsessed with the subject of revenge to the complete exclusion of all other issues in his life.

Epilogue

The first section of this book deals with general concepts of a therapeutic working relationship. Section II attempts to place these concepts in the context of relationship problems between practitioner and patient that are encountered in daily practice. In the necessary interest of space these have been limited to 21 issues submitted to me over the years in which I invited such questions. I am fully aware that we were not able to encompass the entire subject in this limited space, and therefore welcome the opportunity to receive and answer readers' questions through the publisher. Furthermore, I am certain that there are other answers that would enlighten all of us and they are just as welcome.

Notes

[1]

Borderline personality:

Highly disruptive impulsivity, unstable moods and behavior, aggression, self-destructive and negative in all aspects of life including relationships. I see this as a sign of Liver *Qi* deficiency.

Oral personality:

The oral personality is dependent upon others, exceeding the usual parameters in otherwise natural state of affairs, both in degree and kind. Such persons feel inadequate to care for themselves, and at the same time feel that this care should be provided by others. Interpersonal relations are sticky and clinging, marked by demands for succor of all kinds, including financial support. In contrast to the schizophrenic, they are capable of perceiving reality with some accuracy; however, they cannot face it alone, felling totally inadequate to the task. Avoidance thereof leads to a variety of real-life disasters, frequently financial and marital. They have no aim in life except to be cared for, and apart from this do not know what they want. Work records are generally extremely poor, with frequent changes in employment. The deep feelings of inadequacy tend to make them very egocentric, self-centered, and generally unfeeling toward others, whose needs they cannot imagine to be as great as, or taking precedence over, theirs. They are envious of others who are seemingly more competent and are bitter toward those whom they see as stronger and who do not give them enough. The demands are endless, the satisfaction short-lived, and the resentment quickly evoked. In the past they have been classified as 'inadequate' or 'immature' personalities.

[Source: Hammer LI. *Dragon rises—red bird flies*. Seattle, WA: Eastland Press; 2005.]

[2]

Transference is characterized by unconscious redirection of feeling from one person to another. It involves the redirection of feelings and desires and especially of those unconsciously retained from childhood toward a new person.

Counter-transference involves the redirection of a therapist's feelings toward a client and the therapist's emotional entanglement with a client.
[Source: http://en.wikipedia.org/wiki/Transference]

[3]

Split pulse:
A pulse quality in which there appear to be two radical arteries, usually in the middle and sometimes proximal positions. Associated with a preoccupation with death, including suicide, it will disappear with the cessation of the preoccupation with death.

Spinning bean:
A pulse quality that loses its normal pulsation in one position and feels inanimate (in my experience sometimes like a splinter) that implies extreme pain and, even more often, shock (e.g., extreme fright).

References

Section I

Introduction

1 "*Noun*: therapeutic treatment: as **a:** remedial treatment of mental or bodily disorder **b:** an agency (as treatment) designed or serving to bring about rehabilitation or social adjustment" (*Merriam-Webster's Medical Dictionary*. Available from: http://medical.merriam-webster.com/medical/therapy.)
2 Hammer LI. *Dragon rises—red bird flies*. Seattle, WA: Eastland Press; 2005: p. 77.

Chapter 3

1 Sullivan, HS. *The interpersonal theory of psychiatry*. London: Routledge; 2003. See also: Sullivan, HS. *Clinical studies in psychiatry*. New York: WW Norton & Company; 1992.

Chapter 4

1 Reik T. *Listening with the third ear: the inner experience of a psychoanalyst*. New York: Grove Press; 1948.
2 Personal Communication; 1974–1982.
3 Sheldon W. *The varieties of human physique: an introduction to constitutional psychology*. New York: Harpers; 1940.
3a Sheldon W. *Atlas of men*. New York: Macmillan Pub Co; 1970.
4 See, for example, Bridges L. *Face reading in Chinese medicine*. Oxford: Churchill Livingstone; 2003.
5 Personal Communication; 1974–1982.
6 Mar T. *Face reading*. New York: Dadd, Mead and Company; 1970.
7 Beinfeld H, Korngold E. *Between heaven and earth: a guide to Chinese medicine*. New York: Ballantine Books; 1992.

8 American Psychiatric Association. *Diagnostic and statistical manual of mental disorders DSM-IV-TR.* 4th ed. Text revision. Arlington, VA: American Psychiatric Publishing, Inc; 2000.

9 See Rolf IP. *Rolfing.* London: Harper Collins; 1987; also Rolf IP. *Rolfing: reestablishing the natural alignment and structural integration of the human body for vitality and well-being.* Rochester, VT: Healing Arts Press; 1989 and Rolf IP. *Rolfing and physical reality.* Rochester, VT: Healing Arts Press; 1990.

10 Perls FS, Hefferkine R, Goodman P. *Gestalt therapy: excitement and growth in the human personality.* New ed. Gouldsboro, ME: Gestalt Journal Press; 1977.

11 Lowen A. *Bioenergetics: the revolutionary therapy that uses the language of the body to heal the problems of the mind.* London: Penguin/Arkana; 1994.

12 Personal Communication.

13 Reich W. *Character analysis.* New York: Orgone Institute Press; 1949. See also, Reich W. *Character analysis.* 3rd enlarged ed. New York: Farrar, Straus and Giroux; 1980.

14 Bresler DE. *Free yourself from pain.* New York: Simon & Schuster; 1979.

15 Voth H, Nahas G. *How to save your child from drugs.* Forest Dale: Paul S. Eriksson; 1987.

16 Colton, H. *The gift of touch: how physical contact improves communication, pleasure, and health.* New York: Putnam Publishing Group; 1983.

17 Sullivan HS. *The interpersonal theory of psychiatry.* New York: WW Norton; 1953.

18 Hammer LI. *Dragon rises—red bird flies.* Seattle, WA: Eastland Press; 2005.

Chapter 5

1 Peabody F. In: Cousins N. *Anatomy of an illness as perceived by the patient.* New York: WW Norton and Co.; 1964.

Section II

Questions and Answers

1 Hammer LI. *Chinese pulse diagnosis: a contemporary approach.* Seattle, WA: Eastland Press; 2005, p.361.

2 Personal Communication; 1974–1982.

3 Hammer LI. *Dragon rises—red bird flies.* Seattle, WA: Eastland Press; 2005.

4 Hammer LI. *Chinese pulse diagnosis*, op cit., especially Chapter 15.

5 Quiller-Couch AT. *The Oxford Book of English Verse, 1250–1900.* Oxford: Clarendon; 1919.

Index